Core Curriculum for Nephrology Nursing

Sixth Edition

Editor: Caroline S. Counts, MSN, RN, CNN

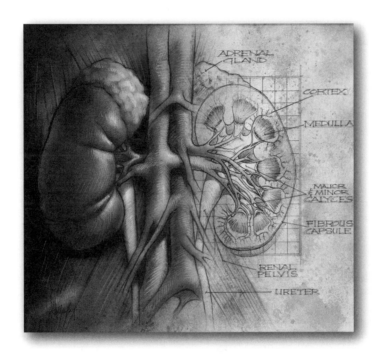

MODULE 5

Kidney Disease in Patient Populations Across the Life Span

ANNA American Nephrology Nurses' Association
www.annanurse.org

Core Curriculum for Nephrology Nursing, 6th Edition

Editor and Project Director
Caroline S. Counts, MSN, RN, CNN

MODULE 5 • Kidney Disease in Patient Populations Across the Life Span

Publication Management
Anthony J. Jannetti, Inc.
East Holly Avenue/Box 56
Pitman, New Jersey 08071-0056

Managing Editor: Claudia Cuddy
Editorial Coordinator: Joseph Tonzelli
Layout Design and Production: Claudia Cuddy
Layout Assistants: Kaytlyn Mroz, Katerina DeFelice, Casey Shea, Courtney Klauber
Design Consultants: Darin Peters, Jack M. Bryant
Proofreaders: Joseph Tonzelli, Evelyn Haney, Alex Grover, Nicole Ward
Cover Design: Darin Peters
Cover Illustration: Scott M. Holladay © 2006
Photography: Kim Counts and Marty Morganello (*unless otherwise credited*)

ANNA National Office Staff
Executive Director: Michael Cunningham
Director of Membership Services: Lou Ann Leary
Membership/Marketing Services Coordinator: Lauren McKeown
Manager, Chapter Services: Janet Betts
Education Services Coordinator: Kristen Kellenyi
Executive Assistant & Marketing Manager, Advertising: Susan Iannelli
Co-Directors of Education Services: Hazel A. Dennison and Sally Russell
Program Manager, Special Projects: Celess Tyrell
Director, Jannetti Publications, Inc.: Kenneth J. Thomas
Managing Editor, *Nephrology Nursing Journal*: Carol Ford
Editorial Coordinator, *Nephrology Nursing Journal:* Joseph Tonzelli
Subscription Manager, *Nephrology Nursing Journal*: Rob McIlvaine
Managing Editor, *ANNA Update, ANNA E-News,* & Web Editor: Kathleen Thomas
Director of Creative Design & Production: Jack M. Bryant
Layout and Design Specialist: Darin Peters
Creative Designer: Bob Taylor
Director of Public Relations and Association Marketing Services: Janet D'Alesandro
Public Relations Specialist: Rosaria Mineo
Vice President, Fulfillment and Information Services: Rae Ann Cummings
Director, Internet Services: Todd Lockhart
Director of Corporate Marketing: Tom Greene
Exhibit Coordinator: Miriam Martin
Conference Manager: Jeri Hendrie
Comptroller: Patti Fortney

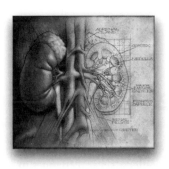

Foreword

The American Nephrology Nurses' Association has had a long-standing commitment to providing the tools and resources needed for individuals to be successful in their professional nephrology roles. With that commitment, we proudly present the sixth edition of the *Core Curriculum for Nephrology Nursing*.

This edition has a new concept and look that we hope you find valuable. Offered in six separate modules, each one will focus on a different component of our specialty and provide essential, updated, high-quality information. Since our last publication of the *Core Curriculum* in 2008, our practice has evolved, and our publication has been transformed to keep pace with those changes.

Under the expert guidance of Editor and Project Director Caroline S. Counts, MSN, RN, CNN (who was also the editor for the 2008 *Core Curriculum*!), this sixth edition continues to build on our fundamental principles and standards of practice. From the basics of each modality to our roles in advocacy, patient engagement, evidence-based practice, and more, you will find crucial information to facilitate the important work you do on a daily basis.

The ANNA Board of Directors and I extend our sincerest gratitude to Caroline and commend her for the stellar work that she and all of the section editors, authors, and reviewers have put forth in developing this new edition of the *Core Curriculum for Nephrology Nursing*. These individuals have spent many hours working to provide you with this important nephrology nursing publication. We hope you enjoy this exemplary professional resource.

Sharon Longton, BSN, RN, CNN, CCTC
ANNA President, 2014-2015

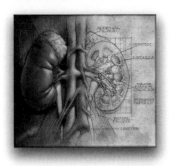

What's new in the sixth edition?

The 2015 edition of the *Core Curriculum for Nephrology Nursing* reflects several changes in format and content. These changes have been made to make life easier for the reader and to improve the scientific value of the *Core*.

1. The *Core Curriculum* is divided into six separate modules that can be purchased as a set or as individual texts. Keep in mind there is likely additional relevant information in more than one module. For example, in Module 2 there is a specific chapter for nutrition, but the topic of nutrition is also addressed in several chapters in other modules.

2. The *Core* is available in both print and electronic formats. The electronic format contains links to other websites with additional helpful information that can be reached with a simple click. With this useful feature comes a potential issue: when an organization changes its website and reroutes its links, the URLs that are provided may not connect. When at the organization's website, use their search feature to easily find your topic. The links in the *Core* were updated as of March 2015.

3. As with the last edition of the *Core*, the pictures on chapter covers depict actual nephrology staff members and patients with kidney disease. Their willingness to participate is greatly appreciated.

4. Self-assessment questions are included at the end of each module for self-testing. Completion of these exercises is not required to obtain CNE. CNE credit can be obtained by accessing the Evaluation Forms on the ANNA website.

5. References are cited in the text and listed at the end of each chapter.

6. We've provided examples of references in APA format at the beginning of each chapter, as well as on the last page of this front matter, to help the readers know how to properly format references if they use citations from the *Core*. The guesswork has been eliminated!

7. The information contained in the *Core* has been expanded, and new topics have been included. For example, there is information on leadership and management, material on caring for Veterans, more emphasis on patient and staff safety, and more.

8. Many individuals assisted in making the *Core* come to fruition; they brought with them their own experience, knowledge, and literature search. As a result, a topic can be addressed from different perspectives, which in turn gives the reader a more global view of nephrology nursing.

9. This edition employs usage of the latest terminology in nephrology patterned after the National Kidney Foundation.

10. The *Core Curriculum for Nephrology Nursing*, 6th edition contains 233 figures, 234 tables, and 29 appendices. These add valuable tools in delivering the contents of the text.

Thanks to B. Braun Medical Inc. for its grant in support of ANNA's *Core Curriculum*.

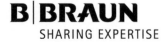

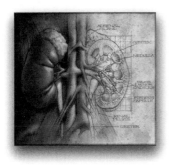

Preface

The sixth edition of the *Core Curriculum for Nephrology Nursing* has been written and published due to the efforts of many individuals. Thank you to the editors, authors, reviewers, and everyone who helped pull the *Core* together to make it the publication it became. A special thank you to Claudia Cuddy and Joe Tonzelli, who were involved from the beginning to the end — I could not have done my job without them!

The overall achievement is the result of the unselfish contributions of each and every individual team member. At times it was a daunting, challenging task, but the work is done, and all members of the "Core-team" should feel proud of the end product.

Now, the work is turned over to you — the reader and learner. I hope you learn at least half as much as I did as pieces of the *Core* were submitted, edited, and refined. Considering the changes that have taken place since the first edition of the *Core* in 1987 (322 pages!), one could say it is a whole new world! Even since the fifth edition in 2008, many changes in nephrology have transpired. This, the 2015 edition, is filled with the latest information regarding kidney disease, its treatment, and the nursing care involved.

But, buyer, beware! Evolution continues, and what is said today can be better said tomorrow. Information continues to change and did so even as the chapters were being written; yet, change reflects progress. Our collective challenge is to learn from the *Core*, be flexible, keep an open mind, and question what could be different or how nephrology nursing practice could be improved.

Nephrology nursing will always be stimulating, learning will never end, and progress will continue! So, the *Core* not only represents what we know now, but also serves as a springboard for what the learner can become and what nephrology nursing can be. A Chinese proverb says this: "Learning is like rowing upstream; not to advance is to drop back."

A final thank-you to the Core-team and a very special note of appreciation to those I love the most. (Those I love the most have also grown since the last edition!) For their love, support, and encouragement, I especially thank my husband, Henry, who thought I had retired; my son and daughter-in law, Chris and Christina, and our two amazing grandchildren, Cate and Olin; and my son-in-law, Marty Morganello, and our daughter, Kim, who provided many of the photographs used in this version of the *Core*. It has been a family project!

Last, but certainly not least, I thank the readers and learners. It is your charge to use the *Core* to grow your minds. Minds can grow as long as we live — don't drop back!

Caroline S. Counts
Editor, Sixth Edition

Module 5

Nephrology nurses take care of patients with kidney disease across the life span. It is possible that the patient is still in the womb or could be quite elderly. This module covers topics that are pertinent to both ends of the life cycle.

In **Chapter 1**, the pediatric chapter, the reader will find useful information on young patients with chronic kidney disease (CKD), complications of CKD in the young, acute kidney injury, treatments with kidney replacement therapies, and the special nutritional and pharmacological needs of the youthful patient. Helping adolescent patients transition to adult care is also addressed.

Chapter 2 focuses on the care of the older adult with kidney disease. The aging process and the care of the older patient with kidney disease are addressed. This is a patient population whose numbers are on the rise. Unless nurses work strictly with pediatric patients, they will be delivering care to elderly patients. The special considerations in caring for this patient population must be taken into account.

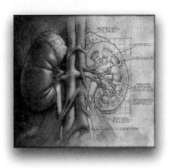

Chapter Editors and Authors

Lisa Ales, MSN, NP-C, FNP-BC, CNN
Clinical Educator, Renal
Baxter Healthcare Corporation
Deerfield, IL
Author: Module 3, Chapter 4

Kim Alleman, MS, APRN, FNP-BC, CNN-NP
Nurse Practitioner
Hartford Hospital Transplant Program
Hartford, CT
Editor: Module 6

Billie Axley, MSN, RN, CNN
Director, Innovations Group
FMS Medical Office
Franklin, TN
Author: Module 4, Chapter 3

Donna Bednarski, MSN, RN, ANP-BC, CNN, CNP
Nurse Practitioner, Dialysis Access Center
Harper University Hospital
Detroit, MI
Editor & Author: Module 1, Chapter 3
Editor & Author: Module 2, Chapter 3
Author: Module 6, Chapter 3

Brandy Begin, BSN, RN, CNN
Pediatric Dialysis Coordinator
Lucile Packard Children's Hospital at Stanford
Palo Alto, CA
Author: Module 5, Chapter 1

Deborah Brommage, MS, RDN, CSR, CDN
Program Director
National Kidney Foundation
New York, NY
Editor & Author: Module 2, Chapter 4
Editor: Module 4, Chapter 3

Deborah H. Brooks, MSN, ANP-BC, CNN, CNN-NP
Nurse Practitioner
Medical University of South Carolina
Charleston, SC
Author: Module 6, Chapter 1

Colleen M. Brown, MSN, APRN, ANP-BC
Transplant Nurse Practitioner
Hartford Hospital
Hartford, CT
Author: Module 6, Chapter 3

Loretta Jackson Brown, PhD, RN, CNN
Health Communication Specialist
Centers for Disease Control and Prevention
Atlanta, GA
Author: Module 2, Chapter 3

Molly Cahill, MSN, RN, APRN, BC, ANP-C, CNN
Nurse Practitioner
KC Kidney Consultants
Kansas City, MO
Author: Module 2, Chapter 3

Sally F. Campoy, DNP, ANP-BC, CNN-NP
Nurse Practitioner, Renal Section
Department of Veterans Affairs
Eastern Colorado Health System
Denver VA Medical Center, Denver, CO
Author: Module 6, Chapter 2

Laurie Carlson, MSN, RN
Transplant Coordinator
University of California –
  San Francisco Medical Center
San Francisco, CA
Author: Module 3, Chapter 1

Deb Castner, MSN, APRN, ACNP, CNN
Nurse Practitioner
Jersey Coast Nephrology & Hypertension
  Associates
Brick, NJ
Author: Module 2, Chapter 3
Author: Module 3, Chapter 2

Louise Clement, MS, RDN, CSR, LD
Renal Dietitian
Fresenius Medical Care
Lubbock, TX
Author: Module 2, Chapter 4

Jean Colaneri, ACNP-BC, CNN
Clinical Nurse Specialist and Nurse
  Practitioner, Dialysis Apheresis
Albany Medical Center Hospital, Albany, NY
Editor & Author: Module 3, Chapter 1

Ann Beemer Cotton, MS, RDN, CNSC
Clinical Dietitian Specialist in Critical Care
IV Health/Methodist Campus
Indianapolis, IN
Author: Module 2, Chapter 4
Author: Module 4, Chapter 2

Caroline S. Counts, MSN, RN, CNN
Research Coordinator, Retired
Division of Nephrology
Medical Unversity of South Carolina
Charleston, SC
Editor: Core Curriculum for Nephrology Nursing
Author: Module 1, Chapter 2
Author: Module 2, Chapter 6
Author: Module 3, Chapter 3

Helen Currier, BSN, RN, CNN, CENP
Director, Renal Services, Dialysis/Pheresis,
  Vascular Access/Wound, Ostomy,
  Continence, & Palliative Care Services
Texas Children's Hospital, Houston, TX
Author: Module 6, Chapter 5

Kim Deaver, MSN, RN, CNN
Program Manager
University of Virginia
Charlottesville, VA
Editor & Author: Module 3, Chapter 3

Anne Diroll, MA, BSN, BS, RN, CNN
Consultant
Volume Management
Rocklin, CA
Author: Module 5, Chapter 1

Daniel Diroll, MA, BSN, BS, RN
Education Coordinator
Fresenius Medical Care North America
Rocklin, CA
Author: Module 2, Chapter 3

Sheila J. Doss-McQuitty, MBA, BSN, RN, CNN, CCRA
Director, Clinical Programs and Research
Satellite Healthcare, Inc., San Jose, CA
Author: Module 2, Chapter 1

Paula Dutka, MSN, RN, CNN
Director, Education and Research
Nephrology Network
Winthrop University Hospital, Mineola, NY
Author: Module 2, Chapter 1

Andrea Easom, MA, MNSc, APRN, FNP-BC, CNN-NP
Instructor, College of Medicine
Nephrology Division
University of Arkansas for Medical Sciences
Little Rock, AR
Author: Module 6, Chapter 2

Rowena W. Elliott, PhD, RN, CNN, CNE, AGNP-C, FAAN
Associate Professor and Chairperson
Department of Advanced Practice
College of Nursing
University of Southern Mississippi
Hattiesburg, MS
Editor & Author: Module 5, Chapter 2

Susan Fallone, MS, RN, CNN
Clinical Nurse Specialist, Retired
Adult and Pediatric Dialysis
Albany Medical Center, Albany, NY
Author: Module 4, Chapter 2

Jessica J. Geer, MSN, C-PNP, CNN-NP
Pediatric Nurse Practitioner
Texas Children's Hospital, Houston, TX
Instructor, Renal Services, Dept. of Pediatrics
Baylor College of Medicine, Houston, TX
Author: Module 6, Chapter 5

Silvia German, RN, CNN
Clinical Writer, CE Coordinator
Manager, DaVita HealthCare Partners Inc.
Denver, CO
Author: Module 2, Chapter 6

Elaine Go, MSN, NP, CNN-NP
Nurse Practitioner
St. Joseph Hospital Renal Center
Orange, CA
Author: Module 6, Chapter 3

Norma Gomez, MSN, MBA, RN, CNN
Nephrology Nurse Consultant
Russellville, TN
Editor & Author: Module 1, Chapter 4

Janelle Gonyea, RDN, LD
Clinical Dietitian
Mayo Clinic
Rochester, MN
Author: Module 2, Chapter 4

Karen Greco, PhD, RN, ANP-BC, FAAN
Nurse Practitioner
Independent Contractor/Consultant
West Linn, OR
Author: Module 2, Chapter 1

Bonnie Bacon Greenspan, MBA, BSN, RN
Consultant, BBG Consulting, LLC
Alexandria, VA
Author: Module 1, Chapter 1

Cheryl L. Groenhoff, MSN, MBA, RN, CNN
Clinical Educator, Baxter Healthcare
Plantation, FL
Author: Module 2, Chapter 3
Author: Module 3, Chapter 4

Debra J. Hain, PhD, ARNP, ANP-BC, GNP-BC, FAANP
Assistant Professor/Lead AGNP Faculty
Florida Atlantic University
Christine E. Lynn College of Nursing
Boca Raton, FL
Nurse Practitioner, Cleveland Clinic Florida
Department of Nephrology, Weston, FL
Editor & Author: Module 2, Chapter 2

Lisa Hall, MSSW, LICSW
Patient Services Director
Northwest Renal Network (ESRD Network 16)
Seattle, WA
Author: Module 2, Chapter 3

Mary S. Haras, PhD, MS, MBA, APN, NP-C, CNN
Assistant Professor and Interim Associate Dean of Graduate Nursing
Saint Xavier University School of Nursing
Chicago, IL
Author: Module 2, Chapter 2

Carol Motes Headley, DNSc, ACNP-BC, RN, CNN
Nephrology Nurse Practitioner
Veterans Affairs Medical Center
Memphis, TN
Editor & Author: Module 2, Chapter 1

Mary Kay Hensley, MS, RDN, CSR
Chair/Immediate Past Chair
Renal Dietitians Dietetic Practice Group
Renal Dietitian, Retired
DaVita HealthCare Partners Inc.
Gary, IN
Author: Module 2, Chapter 4

Kerri Holloway, RN, CNN
Clinical Quality Manager
Corporate Infection Control Specialist
Fresenius Medical Services, Waltham, MA
Author: Module 2, Chapter 6

Alicia M. Horkan, MSN, RN, CNN
Assistant Director, Dialysis Services
Dialysis Center at Colquitt Regional Medical Center
Moultrie, GA
Author: Module 1, Chapter 2

Katherine Houle, MSN, APRN, CFNP, CNN-NP
Nephrology Nurse Practitioner
Marquette General Hospital
Marquette, MI
Editor: Module 6
Author: Module 6, Chapter 3

Liz Howard, RN, CNN
Director
DaVita HealthCare Partners Inc.
Oldsmar, FL
Author: Module 2, Chapter 6

Darlene Jalbert, BSN, RN, CNN
HHD Education Manager
DaVita University School of Clinical Education Wisdom Team
DaVita HealthCare Partners Inc., Denver, CO
Author: Module 3, Chapter 2

Judy Kauffman, MSN, RN, CNN
Manager, Acute Dialysis and Apheresis Unit
University of Virginia Health Systems
Charlottesville, VA
Author: Module 3, Chapter 2

Tamara Kear, PhD, RN, CNS, CNN
Assistant Professor of Nursing
Villanova University, Villanova, PA
Nephrology Nurse, Fresenius Medical Care
Philadelphia, PA
Editor & Author: Module 1, Chapter 2

Lois Kelley, MSW, LSW, ACSW, NSW-C
Master Social Worker
DaVita HealthCare Partners Inc.
Harrisonburg Dialysis
Harrisonburg, VA
Author: Module 2, Chapter 3

Pamela S. Kent, MS, RDN, CSR, LD
Patient Education Coordinator
Centers for Dialysis Care
Cleveland, OH
Author: Module 2, Chapter 4

Carol L. Kinzner, MSN, ARNP, GNP-BC, CNN-NP
Nurse Practitioner
Pacific Nephrology Associates
Tacoma, WA
Author: Module 6, Chapter 3

Kim Lambertson, MSN, RN, CNN
Clinical Educator
Baxter Healthcare
Deerfield, IL
Author: Module 3, Chapter 4

Sharon Longton, BSN, RN, CNN, CCTC
Transplant Coordinator/Educator
Harper University Hospital
Detroit, MI
Author: Module 2, Chapter 3

Maria Luongo, MSN, RN
CAPD Nurse Manager
Massachusetts General Hospital
Boston, MA
Author: Module 3, Chapter 5

Suzanne M. Mahon, DNSc, RN, AOCN, APNG
Professor, Internal Medicine
Division of Hematology/Oncology
Professor, Adult Nursing, School of Nursing
St. Louis University, St. Louis, MO
Author: Module 2, Chapter 1

Nancy McAfee, MN, RN, CNN
CNS – Pediatric Dialysis and Vascular Access
Seattle Children's Hospital
Seattle, WA
Editor & Author: Module 5, Chapter 1

Maureen P. McCarthy, MPH, RDN, CSR, LD
Assistant Professor/Transplant Dietitian
Oregon Health & Science University
Portland, OR
Author: Module 2, Chapter 4

M. Sue McManus, PhD, APRN, FNP-BC, CNN
Nephrology Nurse Practitioner
Kidney Transplant Nurse Practitioner
Richard L. Roudebush VA Medical Center
Indianapolis, IN
Author: Module 1, Chapter 2

Lisa Micklos, BSN, RN
Clinical Educator
NxStage Medical, Inc.
Los Angeles, CA
Author: Module 1, Chapter 2

Michele Mills, MS, RN, CPNP
Pediatric Nurse Practitioner
Pediatric Nephrology
University of Michigan
C.S. Mott Children's Hospital, Ann Arbor, MI
Author: Module 5, Chapter 1

Geraldine F. Morrison, BSHSA, RN
Clinical Director, Home Programs & CKD
Northwest Kidney Center
Seattle, WA
Author: Module 3, Chapter 5

Theresa Mottes, RN, CDN
Pediatric Research Nurse
Cincinnati Children's Hospital & Medical Center
Center for Acute Care Nephrology
Cincinnati, OH
Author: Module 5, Chapter 1

Linda L. Myers, BS, RN, CNN, HP
RN Administrative Coordinator, Retired
Home Dialysis Therapies
University of Virginia Health System
Charlottesville, VA
Author: Module 4, Chapter 5

Clara Neyhart, BSN, RN, CNN
Nephrology Nurse Clinician
UNC Chapel Hill
Chapel Hill, NC
Editor & Author: Module 3, Chapter 1

Mary Alice Norton, BSN, FNP-C
Senior Heart Failure/LVAD/Transplant
    Coordinator
Albany Medical Center Hospital
Albany, NY
Author: Module 4, Chapter 6

Jessie M. Pavlinac, MS, RDN, CSR, LD
Director, Clinical Nutrition
Oregon Health and Science University
Portland, OR
Author: Module 2, Chapter 4

Glenda M. Payne, MS, RN, CNN
Director of Clinical Services
Nephrology Clinical Solutions
Duncanville, TX
Editor & Author: Module 1, Chapter 1
Author: Module 3, Chapter 2
Author: Module 4, Chapter 4

**Eileen J. Peacock, MSN, RN, CNN,
    CIC, CPHQ, CLNC**
Infection Control and Surveillance
    Management Specialist
DaVita HealthCare Partners Inc.
Maple Glen, PA
Editor & Author: Module 2, Chapter 6

Mary Perrecone, MS, RN, CNN, CCRN
Clinical Manager
Fresenius Medical Care
Charleston, SC
Author: Module 4, Chapter 1

Susan A. Pfettscher, PhD, RN
California State University Bakersfield
    Department of Nursing, Retired
Satellite Health Care, San Jose, CA, Retired
Bakersfield, CA
Author: Module 1, Chapter 1

Nancy B. Pierce, BSN, RN, CNN
Dialysis Director
St. Peter's Hospital
Helena, MT
Author: Module 1, Chapter 1

Leonor P. Ponferrada, BSN, RN, CNN
Education Coordinator
University of Missouri School of Medicine –
    Columbia
Columbia, MO
Author: Module 3, Chapter 4

Lillian A. Pryor, MSN, RN, CNN
Clinical Manager
FMC Loganville, LLC
Loganville, GA
Author: Module 1, Chapter 1

Timothy Ray, DNP, CNP, CNN-NP
Nurse Practitioner
Cleveland Kidney & Hypertension Consultants
Euclid, OH
Author: Module 6, Chapter 4

Cindy Richards, BSN, RN, CNN
Transplant Coordinator
Children's of Alabama
Birmingham, AL
Author: Module 5, Chapter 1

Karen C. Robbins, MS, RN, CNN
Nephrology Nurse Consultant
Associate Editor, *Nephrology Nursing Journal*
Past President, American Nephrology Nurses'
    Association
West Hartford, CT
Editor: Module 3, Chapter 2

Regina Rohe, BS, RN, HP(ASCP)
Regional Vice President, Inpatient Services
Fresenius Medical Care, North America
San Francisco, CA
Author: Module 4, Chapter 8

Francine D. Salinitri, PharmD
Associate (Clinical) Professor of
    Pharmacy Practice
Wayne State University, Applebaum College of
    Pharmacy and Health Sciences, Detroit, MI
Clinical Pharmacy Specialist, Nephrology
Oakwood Hospital and Medical Center
Dearborn, MI
Author: Module 2, Chapter 5

Karen E. Schardin, BSN, RN, CNN
Clinical Director, National Accounts
NxStage Medical, Inc.
Lawrence, MA
Editor & Author: Module 3, Chapter 5

Mary Schira, PhD, RN, ACNP-BC
Associate Professor
Univ. of Texas at Arlington – College of Nursing
Arlington, TX
Author: Module 6, Chapter 1

Deidra Schmidt, PharmD
Clinical Pharmacy Specialist
Pediatric Renal Transplantation
Children's of Alabama
Birmingham, AL
Author: Module 5, Chapter 1

Joan E. Speranza-Reid, BSHM, RN, CNN
Clinic Manager
ARA/Miami Regional Dialysis Center
North Miami Beach, FL
Author: Module 3, Chapter 2

Jean Stover, RDN, CSR, LDN
Renal Dietitian
DaVita HealthCare Partners Inc.
Philadelphia, PA
Author: Module 2, Chapter 4

Charlotte Szromba, MSN, APRN, CNNe
Nurse Consultant, Retired
Department Editor, Nephrology Nursing
    Journal
Naperville, IL
Author: Module 2, Chapter 1

Kirsten L. Thompson, MPH, RDN, CSR
Clinical Dietitian
Seattle Children's Hospital, Seattle, WA
Author: Module 5, Chapter 1

Lucy B. Todd, MSN, ACNP-BC, CNN
Medical Science Liaison
Baxter Healthcare
Asheville, NC
Editor & Author: Module 3, Chapter 4

Susan C. Vogel, MHA, RN, CNN
Clinical Manager, National Accounts
NxStage Medical, Inc.
Los Angeles, CA
Author: Module 3, Chapter 5

Joni Walton, PhD, RN, ACNS-BC, NPc
Family Nurse Practitioner
Marias HealthCare
Shelby, MT
Author: Module 2, Chapter 1

Gail S. Wick, MHSA, BSN, RN, CNNe
Consultant
Atlanta, GA
Author: Module 1, Chapter 2

Helen F. Williams, MSN, BSN, RN, CNN
Special Projects – Acute Dialysis Team
Fresenius Medical Care
Denver, CO
Editor: Module 4
Editor & Author: Module 4, Chapter 7

Elizabeth Wilpula, PharmD, BCPS
Clinical Pharmacy Specialist
Nephrology/Transplant
Harper University Hospital, Detroit, MI
Editor & Author: Module 2, Chapter 5

Karen Wiseman, MSN, RN, CNN
Manager, Regulatory Affairs
Fresenius Medical Services
Waltham, MA
Author: Module 2, Chapter 6

Linda S. Wright, DrNP, RN, CNN, CCTC
Lead Kidney and Pancreas Transplant
  Coordinator
Thomas Jefferson University Hospital
Philadelphia, PA
Author: Module 1, Chapter 2

Mary M. Zorzanello, MSN, APRN
Nurse Practitioner, Section of Nephrology
Yale University School of Medicine
New Haven, CT
Author: Module 6, Chapter 3

STATEMENTS OF DISCLOSURE

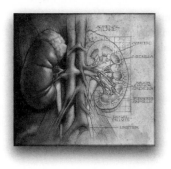

Reviewers

The Blind Review Process

The contents of the *Core Curriculum* underwent a "blind" review process by qualified individuals. One or more chapters were sent to chosen people for critical evaluation. The reviewer did not know the author's identity at the time of the review.

The work could be accepted (1) as originally submitted without revisions, (2) with minor revisons, or (3) with major revisions. The reviewers offered tremendous insight and suggestions; some even submitted additional references they thought might be useful. The results of the review were then sent back to the chapter/module editors to incorporate the suggestions and make revisions.

The reviewers will discover who the authors are now that the *Core* is published. However, while there is this published list of reviewers, no one will know who reviewed which part of the *Core*. That part of the process remains blind.

Because of the efforts of individuals listed below, value was added to the sixth edition. Their hard work is greatly appreciated.

Caroline S. Counts, Editor

Marilyn R. Bartucci, MSN, RN, ACNS-BC, CCTC
Case Manager
Kidney Foundation of Ohio
Cleveland, OH

Christina M. Beale, RN, CNN
Director, Outreach and Education
Lifeline Vascular Access
Vernon Hills, IL

Jenny Bell, BSN, RN, CNN
Clinical Transplant Coordinator
Banner Good Samaritan Transplant Center
Phoenix, AZ

M. Geraldine Biddle, RN, CNN, CPHQ
President, Nephrology Nurse Consultants
Pittsford, NY

Randee Breiterman White, MS, RN
Nurse Case Manager Nephrology
Vanderbilt University Hospital
Nashville, TN

Jerrilynn D. Burrowes, PhD, RDN, CDN
Professor and Chair
Director, Graduate Programs in Nutrition
Department of Nutrition
Long Island University (LIU) Post
Brookville, NY

Sally Burrows-Hudson, MSN, RN, CNN
Deceased 2014
Director, Nephrology Clinical Solutions
Lisle, IL

LaVonne Burrows, APRN, BC, CNN
Advanced Practice Registered Nurse
Springfield Nephrology Associates
Springfield, MO

Karen T. Burwell, BSN, RN, CNN
Acute Dialysis Nurse
DaVita HealthCare Partners Inc.
Phoenix, AZ

Laura D. Byham-Gray, PhD, RDN
Associate Professor and Director
Graduate Programs in Clinical Nutrition
Department of Nutritional Sciences
School of Health Related Professions
Rutgers University
Stratford, NJ

Theresa J. Campbell, DNP, APRN, FNP-BC
Doctor of Nursing Practice
Family Nurse Practitioner
Carolina Kidney Care
Adjunct Professor of Nursing
University of North Caroline at Pembroke
Fayetteville, NC

Monet Carnahan, BSN, RN, CDN
Renal Care Coordinator Program Manager
Fresenius Medical Care
Nashville, TN

Jacke L. Corbett, DNP, FNP-BC, CCTC
Nurse Practitioner
Kidney/Pancreas Transplant Program
University of Utah Health Care
Salt Lake City, UT

Christine Corbett, MSN, APRN, FNP-BC, CNN-NP
Nephrology Nurse Practitioner
Truman Medical Centers
Kansas City, MO

Sandra Corrigan, FNP-BC, CNN
Nurse Practitioner
California Kidney Medical Group
Thousand Oaks, CA

Maureen Craig, MSN, RN, CNN
Clinical Nurse Specialist – Nephrology
University of California Davis Medical Center
Sacramento, CA

Diane M. Derkowski, MA, RN, CNN, CCTC
Kidney Transplant Coordinator
Carolinas Medical Center
Charlotte, NC

Linda Duval, BSN, RN
Executive Director, FMQAI: ESRD Network 13
ESRD Network
Oklahoma City, OK

Damian Eker, DNP, GNP-C
ARNP, Geriatrics & Adult Health
Adult & Geriatric Health Center
Ft. Lauderdale, FL

Elizabeth Evans, DNP
Nephrology Nurse Practitioner
Renal Medicine Associates
Albuquerque, NM

Susan Fallone, MS, RN, CNN
Clinical Nurse Specialist, Retired
Adult and Pediatric Dialysis
Albany Medical Center
Albany, NY

Karen Joann Gaietto, MSN, BSN, RN, CNN
Acute Clinical Service Specialist
DaVita HealthCare Partners Inc.
Tiffin, OH

Deborah Glidden, MSN, ARNP, BC, CNN
Nurse Practitioner
Nephrology Associates of Central Florida
Orlando, FL

**David Jeremiah Grubbs, RN, CDN,
Paramedic, ACLS, PALS, BCLS,
TNCC, NIH**
Clinical Nurse Manager
Crestwood, KY

**Debra J. Hain, PhD, ARNP, ANP-BC,
GNP-BC, FAANP**
Associate Professor/Lead Faculty AGNP Track
Florida Atlantic University
Christine E. Lynn College of Nursing
Boca Raton, FL
Nurse Practitioner, Cleveland Clinic Florida
Department of Nephrology
Weston, FL

Brenda C. Halstead, MSN, RN, AcNP, CNN
Nurse Practitioner
Mid-Atlantic Kidney Center
Richmond and Petersburg, VA

Emel Hamilton, RN, CNN
Director of Clinical Technology
Fresenius Medical Care
Waltham, MA

Mary S. Haras, PhD, MBA, APN, NP-C, CNN
Associate Dean, Graduate Nursing Programs
Saint Xavier University School of Nursing
Chicago, IL

**Malinda C. Harrington, MSN, RN,
FNP-BC, ANCC**
Pediatric Nephrology Nurse Practitioner
Vidant Medical Center
Greenville, NC

Diana Hlebovy, BSN, RN, CHN, CNN
Nephrology Nurse Consultant
Elyria, OH

Sara K. Kennedy, BSN, RN, CNN
UAB Medicine, Kirklin Clinic
Diabetes Care Coordinator
Birmingham, AL

Nadine "Niki" Kobes, BSN, RN
Manager Staff Education/Quality
Fresenius Medical Care – Alaska JV Clinics
Anchorage, AK

Deuzimar Kulawik, MSN, RN
Director of Clinical Quality
DaVita HealthCare Partners Inc.
Westlake Village, CA

Kristin Larson, RN, ANP, GNP, CNN
Clinical Instructor
College of Nursing
Family Nurse Practitioner Program
University of North Dakota
Grand Forks, ND

Deborah Leggett, BSN, RN, CNN
Director, Acute Dialysis
Jackson Madison County General Hospital
Jackson, TN

Charla Litton, MSN, APRN, FNP-BC, CNN
Nurse Practitioner
UHG/Optum
East Texas, TX

Greg Lopez, BSN, RN, CNN
IMPAQ Business Process Manager
Fresenius Medical Care
New Orleans, LA

Terri (Theresa) Luckino, BSN, RN, CCRN
President, Acute Services
RPNT Acute Services, Inc.
Irving, TX

Alice Luehr, BA, RN, CNN
Home Therapy RN
St. Peter's Hospital
Helena, MT

Maryam W. Lyon, MSN, RN, CNN
Education Coordinator
Fresenius Medical Care
Dayton, OH

**Christine Mudge, MS, RN, PNP/CNS,
CNN, FAAN**
Mill Valley, CA

Mary Lee Neuberger, MSN, APRN, RN, CNN
Pediatric Nephrology
University of Iowa Children's Hospital
Iowa City, IA

Jennifer Payton, MHCA, BSN, RN, CNN
Clinical Support Specialist
HealthStar CES
Goose Creek, SC

April Peters, MSN, RN, CNN
Clinical Informatics Specialist
Brookhaven Memorial Hospital Medical Center
Patchogue, NY

David J. Quan, PharmD, BCPS
Health Sciences Clinical Professor of Pharmacy
Clinical Pharmacist, Liver Transplant Services
UCSF Medical Center
San Francisco, CA

Kristi Robertson, CFNP
Nephrology Nurse Practitioner
Nephrology Associates
Columbus, MS

E. James Ryan, BSN, RN, CDN
Hemodialysis Clinical Services Coordinator
Lakeland Regional Medical Center
Lakeland, FL

June Shi, BSN, RN
Vascular Access Coordinator
Transplant Surgery
Medical University of South Carolina
Charleston, SC

Elizabeth St. John, MSN, RN, CNN
Education Coordinator, UMW Region
Fresenius Medical Care
Milwaukee, WI

Sharon Swofford, MA, RN, CNN, CCTC
Transplant Case Manager
OptumHealth
The Villages, FL

Beth Ulrich, EdD, RN, FACHE, FAAN
Senior Partner, Innovative Health Resources
Editor, *Nephrology Nursing Journal*
Pearland, TX

David F. Walz, MBA, BSN, RN, CNN
Program Director
CentraCare Kidney Program
St. Cloud, MN

Gail S. Wick, MHSA, BSN, RN, CNNe
Consultant
Atlanta, GA

Phyllis D. Wille, MS, RN, FNP-C, CNN, CNE
Nursing Faculty
Danville Area Community College
Danville, Il

Donna L. Willingham, RN, CPNP
Pediatric Nephrology Nurse Practitioner
Washington University St. Louis
St. Louis, MO

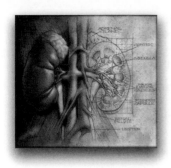

Contents at a Glance

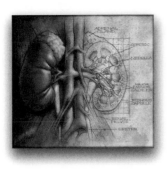

Expanded Contents

The table of contents contains chapters and sections with editors and authors for all six modules. The contents section of this specific module is highlighted in a blue background.

Module 1   Foundations for Practice in Nephrology Nursing

Module 2   Physiologic and Psychosocial Basis for Nephrology Nursing Practice

Module 3   Treatment Options for Patients with Chronic Kidney Failure

Module 4   Acute Kidney Injury

Module 5   Kidney Disease in Patient Populations Across the Life Span

Module 6   The APRN's Approaches to Care in Nephrology

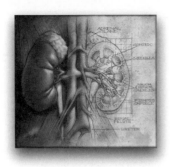

Examples of APA-formatted references

A guide for citing material from Module 5 of the *Core Curriculum for Nephrology Nursing, 6th edition.*

Module 5, Chapter 1

Example of reference for Chapter 1 in APA format. Chapter written by all authors.

McAfee, N., Begin, B., Diroll, A., Mills, M., Mottes, T., Richards, C., Schmidt, D., & Thompson, K.L. (2015). Care of the neonate to adolescent with kidney disease. In C.S. Counts (Ed.), *Core curriculum for nephrology nursing: Module 5. Kidney disease in patient populations across the life span* (6th ed., pp. 1-66). Pitman, NJ: American Nephrology Nurses' Association.

Interpreted: Chapter authors. (Date). Title of chapter. In ...

For citation in text: (McAfee et al., 2015)

Module 5, Chapter 2

Example of reference for Chapter 2 in APA format. One author for entire chapter.

Elliott, R. (2015). Care of the older adult with kidney disease. In C.S. Counts (Ed.), *Core curriculum for nephrology nursing: Module 5. Kidney disease in patient populations across the life span* (6th ed., pp. 67-88). Pitman, NJ: American Nephrology Nurses' Association.

Interpreted: Chapter author. (Date). Title of chapter. In …

For citation in text: (Elliott, 2015)

Care of the Neonate to Adolescent with Kidney Disease

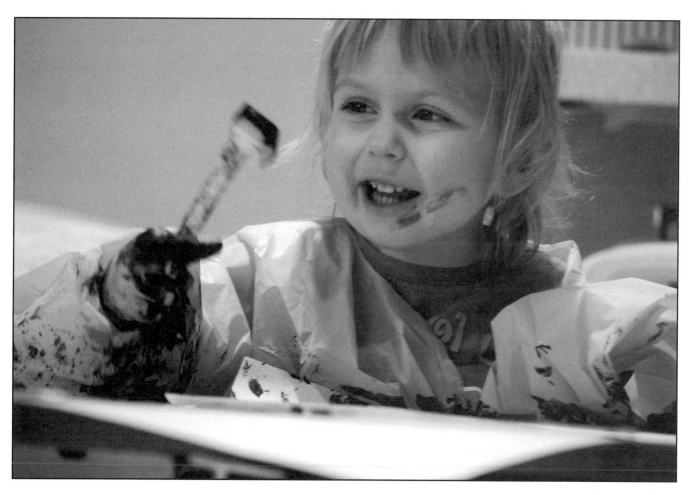

Chapter Editor
Nancy McAfee, MN, RN, CNN

Authors
Nancy McAfee, MN, RN, CNN
Brandy Begin, BSN, RN, CNN
Anne Diroll, MA, BSN, BS, RN, CNN
Michele Mills, MS, RN, CPNP
Theresa Mottes, RN, CDN
Cindy Richards, BSN, RN, CNN
Deidra Schmidt, PharmD
Kirsten L. Thompson, MPH, RDN, CSR

CHAPTER 1

Care of the Neonate to Adolescent with Kidney Disease

This offering for **1.8 contact hours** is provided by the American Nephrology Nurses' Association (ANNA).

American Nephrology Nurses' Association is accredited as a provider of continuing nursing education by the American Nurses Credentialing Center Commission on Accreditation.

ANNA is a provider approved by the California Board of Registered Nursing, provider number CEP 00910.

This CNE offering meets the continuing nursing education requirements for certification and recertification by the Nephrology Nursing Certification Commission (NNCC).

To be awarded contact hours for this activity, read this chapter in its entirety. Then complete the CNE evaluation found at **www.annanurse.org/corecne** and submit it; or print it, complete it, and mail it in. Contact hours are not awarded until the evaluation for the activity is complete.

Example of reference for Chapter 1 in APA format. Chapter written by all authors.

McAfee, N., Begin, B., Diroll, A., Mills, M., Mottes, T., Richards, C., Schmidt, D., & Thompson, K.L. (2015). Care of the neonate to adolescent with kidney disease. In C.S. Counts (Ed.), *Core curriculum for nephrology nursing: Module 5. Kidney disease in patient populations across the life span* (6th ed., pp. 1-66). Pitman, NJ: American Nephrology Nurses' Association.

Interpreted: Chapter authors. (Date). Title of chapter. In ...

Cover photo by Robin Davis, BS, CCLS, Child Life Specialist, Texas Children's Hospital.

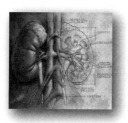

CHAPTER 1

Care of the Neonate to Adolescent with Kidney Disease

Purpose

This chapter outlines the scope and challenges of caring for children from neonate to adolescent who have chronic kidney disease (CKD) stages 1 to 5 or acute kidney injury (AKI). It differentiates their assessment and treatment from the adult care guidelines and assists in preparing and developing clinicians who treat the younger people with kidney disease.

Objectives

Upon completion of this chapter, the learner will be able to:
1. Compare and contrast the systemic effects with the common causes of CKD in children.
2. Discuss the psychosocial impact of CKD on the family.
3. List common causes of acute kidney injury in children.
4. Discuss a child's evaluation for transplantation.
5. Describe challenges to the pediatric patient using hemodialysis, peritoneal dialysis, or continuous renal replacement therapy (CRRT).
6. Explain two specific needs of pediatric patients on hemodialysis (HD).
7. Describe indications for supplemental nutrition in children and identify ways of providing it.

SECTION A
Overview of Pediatric Patients with Chronic Kidney Disease

I. **Kidney disease is a major cause of illness and death in infants, children, and adolescents** (USRDS, 2014).

A. Pediatric patients.
   1. Pediatric patients with CKD, ranging in age from birth to 20 years, are special patients with very special needs.
   2. Their physical and emotional growth relative to their age is often delayed as a consequence of their chronic illness.
   3. On December 31, 2012, 7,522 children were being treated for end-stage renal disease (ESRD). This is a 1.3% decrease in the prevalence of ESRD.
      b. The incident ESRD population declined.
      c. Patients diagnosed as children are transitioned to the adult cohort at the 20th birthday.

B. Incident rate of end-stage renal disease (ESRD) per million in 2012. This is the latest information available at the time of publication (USRDS, 2014).

1. In the United States, the incident rate is 14.1 for children 0 to 19 years old. 1,161 children began treatment for ESRD in 2012.
2. This represents a 5.8% decrease in the incidence of ESRD in this population.
3. The rate is higher for adolescents from 15 to 19 years of age compared to younger ages.
4. Major health consequences of CKD include increased risk of cardiovascular disease as well as kidney failure.

C. Chief causes of CKD in children in the period 2008 to 2012 (USRDS, 2013, 2014).
   1. Cystic/hereditary and congenital disorders account for 35.9% of the incidence of ESRD.
      a. Cystic kidney disease is the most common cause of CKD in children in the United States with a rate that has increased to 5.3 per million people.
      b. In contrast, the rate in Canada is only 0.1, the lowest rate by primary diagnosis (USRDS, 2013).
   2. Glomerular disease caused 21.5% and 10.6% by secondary causes of glomerulonephritis, including vasculitis.
   3. Obstruction/malformations account for 15% to 25% of children with CKD, such as ureteropelvic junction (UPJ) or vesicoureteral junction (VUR).

a. Causes backflow of urine into ureters and possibly kidney pelvis during voiding.
b. Eagle-Barrett or prune belly syndrome (PBS) is a triad of problems including absence of abdominal muscles, urinary tract defects, and cryptorchidism.
c. VATER association is a nonrandom association of anomalies, including:
   (1) V: vertebrae.
   (2) A: anal atresia (there is no opening to the outside of the body).
   (3) TR: tracheoesophageal fistula.
   (4) R: renal anomalies.
   (5) L: often added for limb anomalies (i.e., radial agenesis).

D. Pediatric outcomes from 2007 to 2011 (USRDS, 2013, 2014).
   1. 43.6% transplanted in first year.
   2. 35% of children with CKD stage 5 were readmitted to the hospital within 30 days of a discharge.
   3. Infection rates were highest in youngest patients and those on peritoneal dialysis (PD).
   4. Hospitalizations for bacteremia/sepsis are more frequent in youngest patients.
   5. Hospitalizations for cardiovascular causes from 2007 to 2011:
      a. Decreased 16.8% in children less than 4 years of age.
      b. Rose by 15.6% in ages 5 to 9.
      c. Rose 56.5% in ages 10 to 14.
      d. Increased 31.6% in ages 15 to 19.
      e. Cardiovascular hospitalizations were greatest in the patients on hemodialysis, followed by patients on PD. Patients receiving transplants had the least number of cardiovascular hospitalizations.
   6. Incidence due to cystic/hereditary/congenital diseases is increasing due to earlier diagnosis and treatment.
   7. Children less than 10 years of age appear to be extremely vulnerable to infection, cardiovascular complications, uncontrolled hypertension, and sudden death (USRDS, 2013).

II. Chronic kidney disease is an irreversible deterioration of kidney function that gradually progresses to CKD stage 5 (kidney failure).

A. Both the incidence and progression to CKD stage 5 are equal in both genders, with obstructive uropathies more common in males.
   1. Low birth weight (LBW) babies have a higher risk of CKD (USRDS, 2013).
   2. Despite etiologies, once CKD develops, the failing kidney:
      a. Initially adapts by increasing filtration rate in remaining normal nephrons, a process called adaptive hyperfiltration.
      b. As a result, patients with mild CKD often have a normal or near-normal serum creatinine concentration.
      c. Adaptive hyperfiltration, although initially beneficial, results in long-term damage to the glomeruli of the remaining nephrons.
      d. This is manifested by pathologic proteinuria and progressive kidney insufficiency.
      e. This irreversibility is responsible for the patient's progression to CKD stage 5 when the original illness was thought to be either inactive or cured.
      f. Although the underlying problem that initiated CKD often cannot be treated primarily, extensive studies suggest the progression of the CKD may be due to secondary factors unrelated to initial disease.
         (1) These factors could include anemia, osteodystrophy, systemic and intraglomerular hypertension, glomerular hypertrophy, proteinuria, metabolic acidosis, hyperlipidemia, tubulointerstitial disease, systemic inflammation, and altered prostanoid metabolism.
         (2) This common sequence of events in diverse types of CKD is the basis for common management plans for children with CKD, irrespective of etiology.

B. Pediatric patients.
   1. About 70% of children with chronic kidney disease progress to stage 5 by age 20 years.
   2. Children with CKD stage 5 have a 10-year survival rate of about 80% and an age-specific mortality rate about 30 times than seen in children without kidney failure.
   3. The most common cause of death in these children is cardiovascular disease, followed by infection (USRDS, 2014).
   4. When preemptive transplantation is not an option, the choice between the two forms of dialysis is generally dictated by technical, social, and compliance issues, as well as family preference. Peritoneal dialysis is much more common in infants and younger children (USRDS, 2013).

C. Preemptive kidney transplantation should be the goal in the medical management of children.
   1. Children with CKD and their families should receive education about the following.
      a. The importance of adherence with the treatment plan to prevent secondary complications and natural disease progression.

b. Prescribed medications, highlighting their potential benefits and adverse effects.

c. The prescribed diet.

d. Types of long-term kidney replacement therapies (KRTs).

2. Information related to preemptive kidney transplantation, PD, and hemodialysis should be provided to the family once the child's estimated glomerular filtration rate (eGFR) declines to less than 30 mL/min per 1.73 m² and the child has reached CKD stage 4.

III. History of pediatric nephrology.

A. Through 1940s and 1960s.

1. The focus was on conservative management for CKD such as dietary restrictions, diuretic therapy, electrolyte therapy, and antibacterial use.

2. These interventions offered a shortened critical phase but no long-term improvement (Warady et al., 2004).

B. Beginning in the 1970s.

1 Major university programs began offering end-stage therapy.

2. Conservative therapy was still the most common approach.

3. Children responded differently to dialysis procedures than adults, giving rise to specialized pediatric centers for the treatment of kidney failure (Warady et al., 2004).

C. The 1980s brought widespread use of peritoneal dialysis (PD) modalities.

1. Continuous ambulatory peritoneal dialysis (CAPD) programs for children were begun.

2. Automated systems allowed automated cycling peritoneal dialysis (APD) programs for infants and young children.

3. The early PD access via hard plastic trocar, inserted perpendicular to the abdomen, required complicated maneuvering and propping to keep in position.

4. The hard trocar resulted in complications including intraabdominal injury such as perforation, peritonitis, pain, and discomfort.

5. Introduction of the Tenckhoff® catheter, a less rigid catheter, offered more comfort and options.

6. Dialysate was commercially prepared in large glass bottles that were heavy and required a warming bath to heat.

7. The development of plastic bags for dialysate made home APD possible.

D. The 1990s brought additional advances.

1. Smaller machines with computer technology were developed.

2. Removable data chips allowed transport of treatment details to dialysis centers.

3. Centers were able to remotely download treatment details via modem.

E. Hemodialysis (HD) was initially restricted to adult patients without pediatric equipment available.

1. HD blood lines were cut to create lower volume tubing for pediatric patients.

2. Ultrafiltration (UF) was calculated and transmembrane pressure (TMP) adjusted manually to achieve the desired goal for fluid removal.

3. Small patients required continuous weights to monitor fluid loss.

4. Parallel plate dialyzers increased extracorporeal circuit volume as venous pressure increased and required a higher blood flow rate than most pediatric patients could tolerate.

5. Early dialysis catheters were single lumen that pulled a large volume into the extracorporeal circuit.

6. Acetate dialysate caused frequent emesis.

7. Frequent blood transfusions were required prior to the advent of erythropoiesis-stimulating agents (ESA).

F. Continuous renal replacement therapy (CRRT) modalities in children began in the mid-1980s.

1. Early circuit attempts at continuous arterial-venous hemofiltration (CAVH) required a mean arterial pressure (MAP) of approximately 60 mmHg to move the blood through the circuit. This limited its value for small pediatric patients.

2. Pump systems made it possible to use double lumen venous lines with lower pump speeds.

3. The advent of volumetric systems with integrated blood pump and UF controller finally made the therapy safer for children.

IV. The kidney – a pediatric perspective.

A. Prenatal development.

1. Anatomy and physiology.

a. Urine production begins between 9 and 12 weeks of gestation, contributing to the formation of amniotic fluid.

b. The primary role of the kidneys in utero is development of amniotic fluid which is necessary for pulmonary development.

c. The placenta has the primary responsibility for fluid and electrolyte balance in utero.

d. The development of the nephron continues until 34 to 35 weeks gestation.

e. During the last trimester of pregnancy, there is rapid structural and functional development of the kidneys.

2. Maturational factors that limit kidney function.
   a. Glomerular filtration rate (GFR) is low at birth despite correction for body surface area (BSA).
   b. Kidney blood flow greatly increases during first week of postnatal life.
      (1) At 28 weeks gestational age, the kidney blood flow is 10 mL/min/m².
      (2) By 35 weeks gestational age, the rate is 35 mL/min/m².
   c. Renal tubular immaturity leads to:
      (1) Low capacity to vary sodium and water reabsorption.
      (2) High fractional excretion of sodium (especially in preterm infants).
      (3) Limited ability to concentrate urine.
3. Gestational history.
   a. Oligohydramnios, too little amniotic fluid, suggests:
      (1) Renal agenesis, which is the absence of the ureters, kidneys, and renal arteries.
      (2) Renal hypoplasia (underdevelopment) or dysplasia (developmental or genetic defect with many levels of severity).
      (3) Severe obstruction of urinary tract.
   b. Lack of amniotic fluid around the fetus is responsible for the nonrenal features of Potter's syndrome (malformation or total absence of infant kidneys) including:
      (1) Dysmorphic facies (i.e., altered appearance or facial expressions).
      (2) Aberrant hand and foot positioning.
      (3) Pulmonary hypoplasia (incomplete development of lung tissue).
      (4) Deficient late fetal growth.
   c. Polyhydramnios (too much amniotic fluid) suggests:
      (1) Severe swallowing difficulties caused by neurologic disturbances or upper alimentary tract obstructive disorders.
      (2) Up to 50% of patients with esophageal atresia or tracheoesophageal fistula also have renal malformations.

B. Postnatal development.
   1. Development of the blood flow in the kidneys.
      a. Within 24 hours after birth, the kidney's vascular resistance decreases.
      b. The blood flow rate in the kidneys increases to 15% of the cardiac output.
   2. Development of GFR.
      a. The blood flow to the outer cortical areas increases at 36 weeks.
      b. Positive pressure mechanical ventilation and continuous positive airway pressure (CPAP) can impair the kidney's perfusion.
      c. Nephron formation is complete in term infants.

   d. Preterm infants will continue to develop nephrons until 36 weeks postconception age.
3. Serum creatinine (SCr) concentration.
   a. At birth, the SCr will be equal to the mother's serum creatinine.
   b. In term infants, the serum creatinine falls to 0.4 to 0.5 mg/dL by day 5 to 7.
   c. In preterm infants, the SCr may remain at 1.0 to 1.5 mg/dL for several weeks after birth.
4. Postnatal changes in body fluid composition.
   a. Total body water (TBW) normally decreases after birth related to diuresis (1 to 8 mL/kg/hr).
   b. Diuresis which usually begins within days depends on:
      (1) The degree of excess fluid present at birth.
      (2) The degree of prematurity (more premature infants have greater extracellular fluid [ECF] thus have less diuresis).
      (3) The hemodynamic changes that occur as cardiac output to the kidneys increases and pulmonary circulation opens.
      (4) The decrease in circulating antidiuretic hormone (ADH) levels after delivery.
5. Tubular function.
   a. The functional maturation of the nephron is age rather than body weight dependent.
   b. Increase in tubular length continues until 6 months of age.
   c. The reduced ability of the kidney to reabsorb sodium and water decreases its ability to concentrate urine.
   d. Large amounts of electrolytes and nitrogen are retained to meet growth needs.
   e. Hydrogen ion excretion is reduced for first year of life.
   f. Infants less than 30 weeks of age at birth may develop hyponatremia or hypernatremia due to lower distal tubular reabsorption.
   g. Infants achieve positive potassium (K+) balance within 10 days of birth if fed orally.
   h. Urinary K+ may remain high if formula fed as the body excretes excess K+.

V. Common causes of kidney disease in children.

A. Glomerulonephritis (GN).
   1. Description.
      a. Glomerulonephritis (GN) is a rare but important cause of morbidity and mortality in patients of all ages throughout the world (Beck et al., 2013).
      b. KDIGO published the first guideline that focused on evaluation and treatment of GN (KDIGO, 2012b, http://kdigo.org/home /glomerulonephritis-gn).
      c. GN is inflammation of the glomeruli and can occur acutely or be a chronic problem.

d. Many conditions can cause GN, some known and some unknown.

e. GN can develop a week or two after an infection, (e.g., strep throat, bacterial endocarditis, or a viral infection such as hepatitis).

f. Immune diseases such as lupus, Goodpasture syndrome, or IgA nephropathy can also cause GN.

g. Vasculitis disorders such as polyarteritis or Wegener's granulomatosis can also cause GN.

h. Some conditions such as hypertension, diabetes, and and focal segmental glomerulosclerosis cause scarring of the glomeruli.

2. Presenting characteristics.
   a. Hematuria.
   b. Proteinuria.
   c. Hypertension.
   d. Edema.
   e. Anemia.
   f. Kidney failure.

3. Diagnostic findings:
   a. Urinalysis may show red blood cells and casts, white blood cells, and proteinuria.
   b. Blood urea nitrogen (BUN) and creatinine elevations.
   c. Kidney biopsy to confirm diagnosis.

B. Nephrotic syndrome (NS).

1. Description.
   a. Nephrotic syndrome can result from primary glomerular disease (idiopathic) or secondary diseases such as systemic lupus erythematosus.
   b. Idiopathic nephrotic syndrome affects 16 in 100,000 children, making this condition one of the more common childhood kidney diseases (Gipson et al., 2014).
   c In a study from 1967 to 1974, of 521 children with nephrotic syndrome, 77% had minimal change nephrotic syndrome (MCNS), 8% had focal segmental glomerulonephritis (FSGS), 6% had membranoproliferative glomerulo-nephritis, and 9% had other underlying causes.
   d. Childhood NS can occur at any age but most commonly between 18 months and 5 years.
   e. Affects males more often than females.
   f. Needs careful evaluation to rule out symptoms as secondary condition (Gipson et al., 2014).

2. Presenting characteristics.
   a. Proteinuria (> 3.5 g/24 hr) (KDOQI, 2012).
   b. Hypoproteinemia < 2.5 mg/dL.
   c. Edema.
   d. Decreased urination.
   e. Weight gain.
   f. Hyperlipidemia.
   g. Lipiduria (lipids in the urine).

3. Diagnostic findings.
   a. Hypoproteinemia (from decreased osmotic pressure in the blood) resulting in edema.
   b. Proteinuria may be asymptomatic; presents during routine health screening.
   c. Proteinuria may be identified as a complicating factor within another health condition.

4. Potential treatments.
   a. Steroid responsive nephrotic syndrome will demonstrate a resolution of proteinuria within 4 weeks of daily therapy.
   b. Frequently relapsing nephrotic syndrome may require extended dosing of glucocorticoids, cytotoxic agents, mycophenolate mofetil, or calcineurin inhibitors.
   c. Treatment is nephrectomy and institution of dialysis when unable to control proteinuria and edema.

5. Associated conditions.
   a. Minimal change disease (Vivante et al., 2014).
   b. Focal segmental glomerulosclerosis (FSGS).
   c. Membranoproliferative glomerulonephritis (MPGN).
   d. Poststreptococcal glomerulonephritis (PSGN).

C. Immune globulin A nephropathy (IgA).

1. Description.
   a. IgA (a protein that helps the body fight infections) settles in the kidneys.
   b. The deposits cause the kidneys to leak blood and protein in the urine.
   c. Excessive protein leak causes edema.
   d. Only 5% to 10% of children develop kidney failure.
   e. More males are affected than females.

2. Presenting characteristics.
   a. Edema.
   b. Nausea.
   c. Fatigue.
   d. Headaches.
   e. Sleep problems.
   f. Hypertension.

3. Diagnostic tests.
   a. Urinalysis to test for blood or protein.
   b. Casts in urine.
   c. BUN and creatinine levels.
   d. Kidney biopsy.

D. Renal tubular acidosis (RTA).

1. Description.
   a. Renal tubular acidosis (RTA) occurs when the kidneys fail to excrete acids, causing acidic buildup in the blood.
   b. Type 1 RTA.
      (1) Classical distal RTA.
      (2) May be inherited as a primary disorder.
      (3) Or, may be the result of autoimmune disorders (such as Sjögren's syndrome or lupus) that attack the distal tubule.

c. Type 2 RTA.
  (1) Also called proximal RTA.
  (2) Occurs most frequently in children as part of Fanconi syndrome.
2. Presenting characteristics.
  a. Hypokalemia or hyperkalemia.
  b. Growth failure.
  c. Kidney stones.
  d. Progressive kidney and bone disease.
  e. Vitamin D deficiency.
3. Diagnostic findings.
  a. Hypokalemia, which may be severe.
  b. Growth failure.
  c. Kidney stones.
  d. Untreated classical distal RTA causes growth retardation in children and progressive kidney and bone disease in adults.
  e. If RTA is suspected, sodium, potassium, and chloride levels in the urine and serum potassium level will help identify the type of RTA.
4. Restoring normal growth and preventing kidney stones are the major goals of therapy.
5. Associated conditions.
  a. Other diseases and conditions associated with classical distal RTA.
    (1) Sickle cell anemia.
    (2) Hyperparathyroidism.
    (3) Hyperthyroidism.
    (4) Chronic active hepatitis.
    (5) Primary biliary cirrhosis.
    (6) A hereditary form of deafness.
    (7) Analgesic nephropathy.
    (8) Rejection of a transplanted kidney.
    (9) Renal medullary cystic disease.
    (10) Obstructive uropathy.
    (11) Chronic urinary tract infections.
  b. Autoimmune disorders, like Sjögren's syndrome and lupus, which also attack the distal tubule.
  c. Proximal RTA.
    (1) Can also result from inherited disorders that disrupt the body's normal breakdown and use of nutrients.
    (2) Examples.
      (a) The rare disease cystinosis, in which cystine crystals are deposited in bones and other tissues.
      (b) Hereditary fructose intolerance.
      (c) Wilson disease.
  d. Proximal RTA also occurs in patients treated with ifosfamide.

E. Fanconi syndrome (Igarashi, 2009).
  1. Description.
    a. Fanconi syndrome is a generalized dysfunction that affects the proximal renal tubules of the kidney.
    b. The condition interferes with the renal tubules'

ability to reabsorb amino acids, glucose, uric acid, bicarbonates, and phosphates, resulting in abnormally low plasma levels.
    c. The causes of Fanconi syndrome are hereditary, acquired, or exogenous substances.
  2. Presenting characteristics.
    a. Growth failure.
    b. Dehydration and excessive thirst.
    c. Muscle weakness and cramping.
    d. Fatigue.
    e. Bone and joint pain.
    f. Recurrent fevers.
  3. Diagnostic findings.
    a. Proteinuria.
    b. Hypokalemia.
    c. Hypophosphatemia.
    d. Hyperchloremic metabolic acidosis.
    e. Abnormal urine electrolytes.
    f. Bone abnormalities.

F. Bartter Syndrome (Devuyst et al., 2009).
  1. Description.
    a. Bartter syndrome is an inherited disorder, altering the reabsorption abilities of the renal tubules.
    b. Bartter is classified according to the specific defect; type I to V.
    c. The severity and presentation differs with each type.
    d. Prevalence is 1 in every 1,000,000.
  2. Presenting characteristics.
    a. Growth failure.
    b. Developmentally delayed.
    c. Polyuria and polydipsia.
    d. Lower blood pressure.
  3. Diagnostic findings.
    a. Abnormal urine electrolytes (calcium, potassium, magnesium).
    b. Hypercalciuria.
    c. Hypocalcemia.
    d. Mild hypomagnesaemia.
    e. Hypokalemia.
    f. Metabolic alkalosis.

G. Gitelman Syndrome (Devuyst et al., 2009).
  1. Description.
    a. Gitelman syndrome is an inherited defect of the renal tubule system.
    b. It causes the kidney to waste magnesium, sodium, potassium, and chloride in the urine, instead of reabsorbing it back into the bloodstream.
    c. Prevalence equals 1 in every 40,000.
  2. Presenting characteristics.
    a. Muscle weakness and cramping.
    b. Fatigue.
    c. Thirst.

d. Paresthesia (numbness).
e. Lower blood pressure.
3. Diagnostic findings.
a. Hypokalemia.
b. Hypomagnesaemia.
c. Hypocalcemia.
d. Abnormal urine electrolytes (calcium, potassium, magnesium).
e. Hypocalciuria.
f. Metabolic alkalosis.

H. Liddle syndrome (Devuyst et al., 2009).
1. Description.
a. Liddle syndrome is a rare genetic disorder of the renal distal tubule that specifically affects sodium reabsorption.
b. Liddle syndrome generally presents at a young age, usually before adolescence.
2. The presenting characteristic is hypertension.
3. Diagnostic findings.
a. Hypokalemia.
b. Metabolic alkalosis.

I. Cystinosis (Gahl, 2009).
1. Description.
a. Cystinosis is an inherited metabolic disease that results in excessive cystine levels in multiple organs and leads to severe organ damage.
b. Divided into three categories.
(1) Infantile is the most severe form and accounts for 95% of cases.
(2) Intermediate is a milder form of the disease and is diagnosed in early adolescence or young adulthood.
(3) Ocular is the rarest and mildest form with minimal symptoms.
c. The infantile and intermediate categories eventually result in CKD.
d. Prevalence is 1 of every 100,000 to 200,000.
2. Presenting characteristics.
a. Polyuria, as much as 2 to 3 L/day.
b. Polydipsia.
c. Weakness.
d. Episodes of dehydration.
e. Unexplained fever.
f. Growth failure/retardation.
g. Tetany.
h. Salt cravings.
i. Blonde hair and pale skin color.
j. Hepatomegaly.
3. Diagnostic findings.
a. Glucosuria.
b. Proteinuria.
c. Hyperchloremic metabolic acidosis.
d. Hypokalemia.
e. Hypouricemia.
f. Elevated intraleukocyte cystine content.

J. Pyelonephritis/malformations of urinary tract.
1. Description.
a. Obstruction of the ureteropelvic junction (UPJ) or vesicoureteral junction (VUR) causes backflow of urine into ureters and possibly the pelvis of the kidney during urination.
b. Eagle-Barrett or prune belly syndrome (PBS) is a triad of problems including absence of abdominal muscles, urinary tract defects, and cryptorchidism.
c. VATER association is a nonrandom association of anomalies, including vertebral defects, anal atresia, tracheoesophageal fistula with esophageal atresia, radial, and kidney defects.
2. The outcome depends on when the malformation occurs in fetal development and the severity of the obstruction.

K. Hereditary disorders.
1. Polycystic kidney disease (PKD).
a. Autosomal recessive polycystic kidney disease (ARPKD) is an inherited disorder involving cystic dilation of the kidney's collecting ducts and varying degrees of hepatic abnormalities consisting of biliary dysgenesis and periportal fibrosis.
(1) The biliary dysgenesis is characterized by proliferation of abnormally shaped ducts in the portal tracts of the liver. The portal tracts contain branches of the hepatic artery and portal vein, the tributaries of the bile duct, and lymphatics.
(2) Periportal fibrosis is due to the formation of excess connective tissue within the portal tracts.
b. Autosomal dominant polycystic kidney disease (ADPKD) is characterized by the presence of cysts at any point along the nephron or collecting duct. It is rarely a significant neonatal presentation but can present with same complications of ARPKD.
2. Alport's syndrome.
a. Description.
(1) An inherited disorder characterized by progressive familial glomerulonephropathy with or without accompanying nerve deafness and ocular abnormalities.
(2) Both males and females are affected. However, the disease is more severe in males.
b. Presenting characteristics.
(1) Hematuria with or without proteinuria.
(2) Gradual progression to kidney failure in late teens or later.

L. Hemolytic uremic syndrome (HUS).
1. Description.
http://kidney.niddk.nih.gov/kudiseases/pubs/child
kidneydiseases/hemolytic_uremic_syndrome/
   a. Shiga-like toxin producing *E. coli* hemolytic-
uremic syndrome (STEC-HUS) usually occurs
when an infection in the digestive system
produces toxic substances that destroy red
blood cells, causing kidney injury.
   b. Characterized by hemolytic anemia,
thrombocytopenia, and acute kidney failure.
   c. It is an acquired disease.
   d. Secondary to endothelial toxicity of infectious
agents, mainly *E. coli* 0157H:7.
   e. It is most common in children < 3 years old.
   f. The mortality rate is < 5%.
   g. There is a 30% risk of kidney sequela.
   h. Rarely relapses.
   i. Low risk of recurrence posttransplant.
2. Presenting characteristics.
   a. Diarrhea positive in 90% of cases.
   b. Bloody diarrhea.
   c. Vomiting.
   d. Abdominal pain.
   e. Pale skin tone.
   f. Fatigue and irritability.
   g. Small, unexplained bruises or bleeding from
the nose and mouth.
   h. Decreased urination or blood in the urine.
   i. Edema.
   j. Confusion.
3. Diagnostic findings.
   a. Thrombocytopenia.
   b. Anemia.
   c. Elevated creatinine.
   d. Hematuria.

M. Atypical HUS (aHUS).
1. Description. http://atypicalhus.net/
   a. aHUS is a rare disease characterized by
hemolytic anemia, thrombocytopenia, and
acute kidney failure.
   b. It is not caused by an external agent.
   c. Does not usually present with diarrhea.
   d. It can affect any age including newborns.
   e. May be familial (either autosomal dominant or
recessive).
   f. It frequently has a recurrent course.
   g. The kidney's prognosis is poor.
   h. Posttransplant recurrence is seen in 30% of
cases.
2. Presenting characteristics.
   a. Vomiting.
   b. Abdominal pain.
   c. Pale skin tone.
   d. Fatigue and irritability.

   e. Small, unexplained bruises or bleeding from
the nose and mouth.
   f. Decreased urination or blood in the urine.
   g. Edema.
   h. Confusion.
   i. Acute kidney injury.
3. Diagnostic findings.
   a. Serum C3 and C4 concentrations may indicate
complement activation or dysregulation.
   b. Thrombocytopenia.
   c. Anemia.

N. Henoch-Schönlein purpura (HSP) (McCarthy, 2010).
1. Description.
   a. Inflammation and bleeding in the small blood
vessels in the skin, joints, intestines, and
kidneys.
   b. Petechial, purpuric rash, predominantly on the
lower extremities.
2. Presenting characteristics.
   a. Purpura.
   b. Swollen, sore joints (arthritis).
   c. Abdominal pain.
   d. Nausea.
   e. Vomiting or bloody stools.
   f. Proteinuria.
   g. Hematuria.
   h. Arthralgias, frequently in lower extremity
joints, are accompanied by periarticular soft
tissue edema.
   i. Petechial or purpuric rash, accompanied by one
of the following.
      (1) Abdominal pain.
      (2) Joint pain.
      (3) Antibody deposits on the skin.
      (4) Hematuria or proteinuria.

SECTION B
Chronic Kidney Disease in Children

I. **Assessment of kidney structure and
function in CKD.**

A. History and physical.
1. The approach used to obtain a health history and
perform a physical examination varies according
to the age of the child.
2. Developmental age-appropriate care is outlined in
Table 1.1.
3. Providing preventive advice or anticipatory
guidance for the parents is an important
component of providing care.

Table 1.1

Developmental Age-Appropriate Care: Preparation/Education/Activity

Developmental Age	Nursing Interventions
0–12 months (infant)	• Support parents' ability to calm/comfort infant by providing parent(s) with adequate information and preparation to reduce their own anxiety. • Provide opportunities for the parent(s) to hold the infant.
12–24 months (toddler)	• Support parents' ability to calm/comfort toddler by providing parent(s) with adequate information and preparation to reduce their own anxiety. • Encourage parent(s) to involve toddler in developmentally appropriate scheduled activities. • Whenever safe and possible, allow toddler to handle items used in his/her care (e.g., blood pressure cuff, face mask). • Offer suggestions to parent(s) about helpful distractions during procedures. If parent(s) are unavailable, offer comfort and/or distraction as appropriate. • Stoop to the child's eye level (face-to-face) and speak softly and calmly.
2–3 years (toddler)	• Support parents ability to calm and comfort toddler by providing parent(s) with adequate information and preparation to reduce their own anxiety. • Encourage parents to use age-appropriate activity areas when available. Activity areas can include a playroom, playground, garden, library, school room, and/or teen room. • Actively involve child in treatment. Whenever safe, allow child to handle/examine equipment used in treatments/procedures. • Provide comfort and/or distraction during tests and procedures. Preparation should begin immediately preceding the event. • Give the child simple explanations of tests and procedures, using the sensory approach (i.e., what child will see, hear, taste, feel). • Provide choices whenever possible (e.g., examine eyes or ears first). • Stoop to the child's eye level (face-to-face) and speak softly and calmly.
3–5 years (preschooler)	• Be honest. • Actively involve child in treatment. • Whenever safe, allow child to handle and explore medical equipment prior to use (e.g., peritoneal dialysis catheter). • Provide comfort and/or distraction during and after tests and procedures. • Use interventions that preserve the child's concept of body integrity (e.g., child-friendly bandages for venipuncture sites).

Continues on next page

B. Developmental age-appropriate care.
  1. Growth and development are continuous dynamic processes involving genetics, nutrition, physical, and psychological factors.
  2. Privacy is important to children.
    a. Adolescents have a growing need for privacy and an opportunity to discuss their growing sexuality, or lack thereof.
    b. Discussions must take place about safe sexual practices and possible birth control. Many may not have a primary care provider (PCP).
  3. Play therapy can facilitate trust, especially for younger children.
    a. Children are often able to verbalize more while involved in play.
    b. Use opportunities while playing to ask questions about the child's understanding of illness, diet, therapy options, etc.
  4. Child life specialists can play a vital supporting role in a dialysis clinic or unit.
    a. These trained specialists use play, biofeedback, and distraction during painful or uncomfortable procedures.
    b. Some children can learn self-calming techniques for coping.
  5. Standardized norms are used for comparison to other children at same age.
    a. Weight is measured and plotted on a standardized growth chart at each visit. The child should follow a standardized growth curve.

Table 1.1 (continued) ———— **Developmental Age-Appropriate Care: Preparation/Education/Activity**

3–5 years (preschooler) (continued from previous page)	• Give the child short, simple explanations of tests and procedures using the sensory approach (e.g., what child will see, hear, taste, feel). Ask for feedback. • Preparation should be done far enough in advance for child to process information, but not too far in advance so that child has time to fantasize — preferably a few hours before the test or procedure. • Encourage child to participate in age-appropriate activities. • Provide choices whenever possible (e.g., which ear to examine first). • Stoop to or sit at the child's eye level (face-to-face) and speak softly and calmly.
6–9 years (school-age)	• Be honest. • Encourage choices among options if possible (e.g., IV in right or left hand for the patient on peritoneal dialysis receiving IV medication therapy). • Whenever safe, allow child to handle and explore medical equipment before use. • Provide comfort and/or distraction during and after tests or procedures. • Give the child developmentally appropriate explanations of tests and procedures using the sensory approach (e.g., what child will see, hear, taste, feel). Ask for feedback. • Preparation should be done far enough in advance for child to process information, but not too far in advance so that child has time to fantasize. • Encourage child to participate in age-appropriate activities. • Provide choices whenever possible (e.g., which limb for venipuncture).
9–12 years (preteen)	• Provide honest and accurate information about potential tests and procedures/treatments, etc. Ask for feedback about what the preteen understands. • Provide developmentally appropriate explanations using the sensory approach (e.g., what the patient will see, hear, feel, etc.). • Provide comfort and/or distraction as needed during procedures that may be uncomfortable or painful. • Encourage participation in decision making whenever possible. • Be clear about what expectations are in terms of learning and self-care/adherence. • Preparation should be done far enough in advance for child to process information. • Provide choices whenever possible (e.g., choices that lead to having some control, such as the preteen having the option of applying tape).
13–18 years (adolescent)	• Provide rationale for treatment. Get feedback regarding adolescent's understanding of tests, procedures, disease process, and treatment plans. • Encourage adolescents to take responsibility for aspect of self-care. Provide positive reinforcement for successes. • It is important to prepare adolescent for what he/she will see, hear, feel, taste, smell, and be expected to do.

b. Height should be measured at least quarterly and plotted on a standardized growth chart (see Figures 1.1 and 1.2).

c. Head circumference is recorded routinely until age 3 years.

d. Failure to thrive or grow on dialysis may indicate an urgent need for transplantation.

e. Respiratory rate, pulse, and temperature are recorded at each visit.

f. Blood pressure (BP) (see Tables 1.2 and 1.3).

g. Annual measurements should be recorded on all children 3 years of age and older. If there is known kidney disease, the BP should be measured at an earlier age.

   (1) An appropriate size cuff is necessary to obtain an accurate reading.

   (2) The cuff width should be 40% of midarm circumference.

   (3) The cuff bladder should cover 80% to 100% of the arm circumference and approximately two thirds the length of upper arm.

   (4) A cuff that is too small will result in a falsely elevated blood pressure reading.

   (5) Measurement should be performed with a sphygmomanometer or a calibrated aneroid device with the child sitting and his or her right arm resting on a solid supporting surface at heart level.

   (6) Blood pressure measurements in

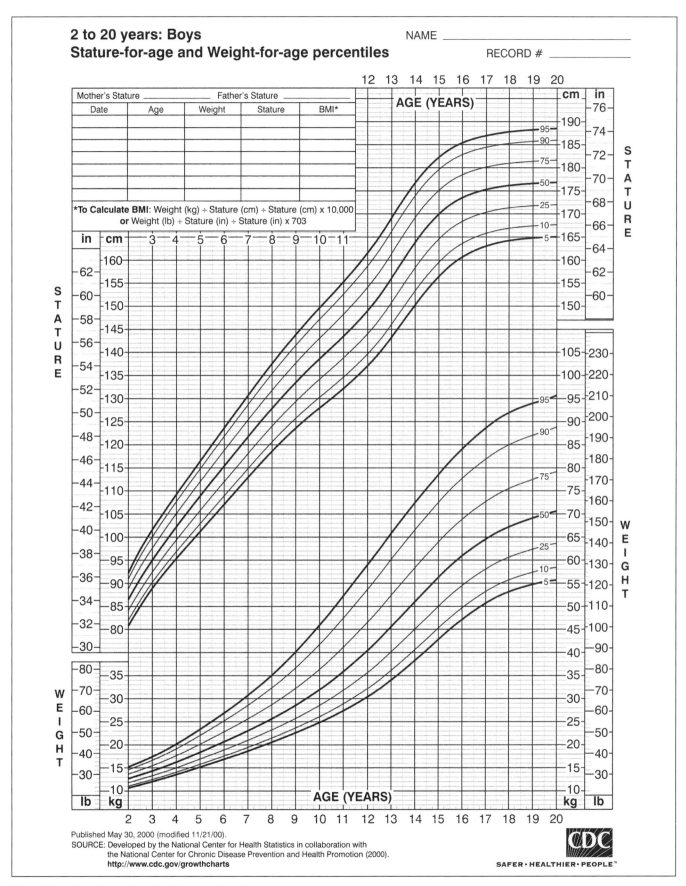

Figure1.1. Growth velocity chart for boys 2 to 20 years.

Source: Centers for Disease Control (2014). http://www.cdc.gov/growthcharts/clinical_charts.htm

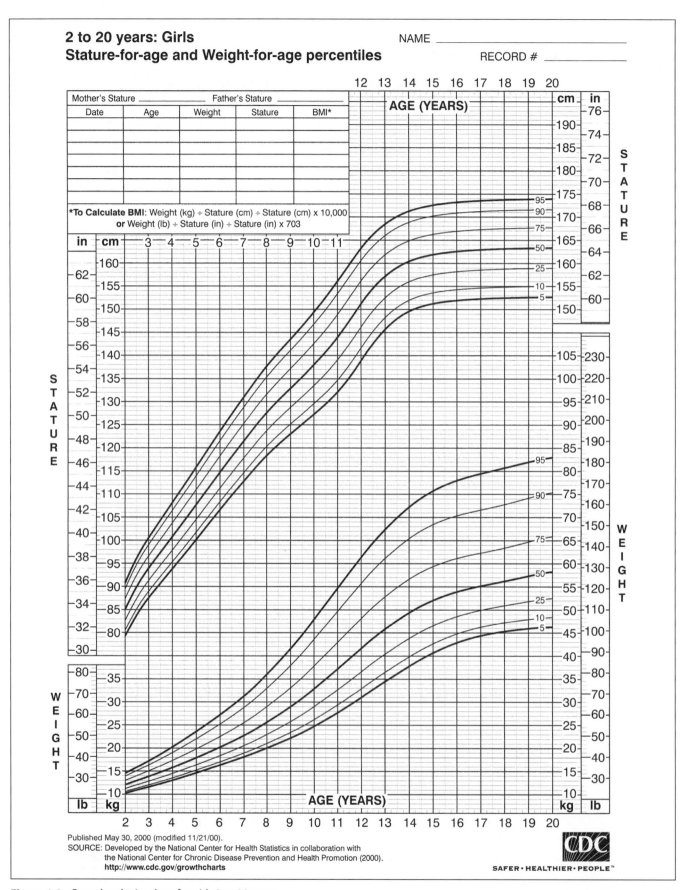

Figure 1.2. Growth velocity chart for girls 2 to 20 years.

Source: Centers for Disease Control (2014). http://www.cdc.gov/growthcharts/clinical_charts.htm

Table 1.2

Blood Pressure Levels for Boys by Age and Height Percentile

Age (Year)	BP Percentile ↓	Systolic BP (mmHg) ← Percentile of Height →							Diastolic BP (mmHg) ← Percentile of Height →						
		5th	10th	25th	50th	75th	90th	95th	5th	10th	25th	50th	75th	90th	95th
1	50th	80	81	83	85	87	88	89	34	35	36	37	38	39	39
	90th	94	95	97	99	100	102	103	49	50	51	52	53	53	54
	95th	98	99	101	103	104	106	106	54	54	55	56	57	58	58
	99th	105	106	108	110	112	113	114	61	62	63	64	65	66	66
2	50th	84	85	87	88	90	92	92	39	40	41	42	43	44	44
	90th	97	99	100	102	104	105	106	54	55	56	57	58	58	59
	95th	101	102	104	106	108	109	110	59	59	60	61	62	63	63
	99th	109	110	111	113	115	117	117	66	67	68	69	70	71	71
3	50th	86	87	89	91	93	94	95	44	44	45	46	47	48	48
	90th	100	101	103	105	107	108	109	59	59	60	61	62	63	63
	95th	104	105	107	109	110	112	113	63	63	64	65	66	67	67
	99th	111	112	114	116	118	119	120	71	71	72	73	74	75	75
4	50th	88	89	91	93	95	96	97	47	48	49	50	51	51	52
	90th	102	103	105	107	109	110	111	62	63	64	65	66	66	67
	95th	106	107	109	111	112	114	115	66	67	68	69	70	71	71
	99th	113	114	116	118	120	121	122	74	75	76	77	78	78	79
5	50th	90	91	93	95	96	98	98	50	51	52	53	54	55	55
	90th	104	105	106	108	110	111	112	65	66	67	68	69	69	70
	95th	108	109	110	112	114	115	116	69	70	71	72	73	74	74
	99th	115	116	118	120	121	123	123	77	78	79	80	81	81	82
6	50th	91	92	94	96	98	99	100	53	53	54	55	56	57	57
	90th	105	106	108	110	111	113	113	68	68	69	70	71	72	72
	95th	109	110	112	114	115	117	117	72	72	73	74	75	76	76
	99th	116	117	119	121	123	124	125	80	80	81	82	83	84	84
7	50th	92	94	95	97	99	100	101	55	55	56	57	58	59	59
	90th	106	107	109	111	113	114	115	70	70	71	72	73	74	74
	95th	110	111	113	115	117	118	119	74	74	75	76	77	78	78
	99th	117	118	120	122	124	125	126	82	82	83	84	85	86	86
8	50th	94	95	97	99	100	102	102	56	57	58	59	60	60	61
	90th	107	109	110	112	114	115	116	71	72	72	73	74	75	76
	95th	111	112	114	116	118	119	120	75	76	77	78	79	79	80
	99th	119	120	122	123	125	127	127	83	84	85	86	87	87	88
9	50th	95	96	98	100	102	103	104	57	58	59	60	61	61	62
	90th	109	110	112	114	115	117	118	72	73	74	75	76	76	77
	95th	113	114	116	118	119	121	121	76	77	78	79	80	81	81
	99th	120	121	123	125	127	128	129	84	85	86	87	88	88	89
10	50th	97	98	100	102	103	105	106	58	59	60	61	61	62	63
	90th	111	112	114	115	117	119	119	73	73	74	75	76	77	78
	95th	115	116	117	119	121	122	123	77	78	79	80	81	81	82
	99th	122	123	125	127	128	130	130	85	86	86	88	88	89	90

The Fourth Report on the Diagnosis, Evaluation, and Treatment of High Blood Pressure in Children and Adolescents

Continues on next page

Table 1.2 (continued)

Blood Pressure Levels for Boys by Age and Height Percentile

Age (Year)	BP Percentile ↓	Systolic BP (mmHg) ← Percentile of Height →							Diastolic BP (mmHg) ← Percentile of Height →						
		5th	10th	25th	50th	75th	90th	95th	5th	10th	25th	50th	75th	90th	95th
11	50th	99	100	102	104	105	107	107	59	59	60	61	62	63	63
	90th	113	114	115	117	119	120	121	74	74	75	76	77	78	78
	95th	117	118	119	121	123	124	125	78	78	79	80	81	82	82
	99th	124	125	127	129	130	132	132	86	86	87	88	89	90	90
12	50th	101	102	104	106	108	109	110	59	60	61	62	63	63	64
	90th	115	116	118	120	121	123	123	74	75	75	76	77	78	79
	95th	119	120	122	123	125	127	127	78	79	80	81	82	82	83
	99th	126	127	129	131	133	134	135	86	87	88	89	90	90	91
13	50th	104	105	106	108	110	111	112	60	60	61	62	63	64	64
	90th	117	118	120	122	124	125	126	75	75	76	77	78	79	79
	95th	121	122	124	126	128	129	130	79	79	80	81	82	83	83
	99th	128	130	131	133	135	136	137	87	87	88	89	90	91	91
14	50th	106	107	109	111	113	114	115	60	61	62	63	64	65	65
	90th	120	121	123	125	126	128	128	75	76	77	78	79	79	80
	95th	124	125	127	128	130	132	132	80	80	81	82	83	84	84
	99th	131	132	134	136	138	139	140	87	88	89	90	91	92	92
15	50th	109	110	112	113	115	117	117	61	62	63	64	65	66	66
	90th	122	124	125	127	129	130	131	76	77	78	79	80	80	81
	95th	126	127	129	131	133	134	135	81	81	82	83	84	85	85
	99th	134	135	136	138	140	142	142	88	89	90	91	92	93	93
16	50th	111	112	114	116	118	119	120	63	63	64	65	66	67	67
	90th	125	126	128	130	131	133	134	78	78	79	80	81	82	82
	95th	129	130	132	134	135	137	137	82	83	83	84	85	86	87
	99th	136	137	139	141	143	144	145	90	90	91	92	93	94	94
17	50th	114	115	116	118	120	121	122	65	66	66	67	68	69	70
	90th	127	128	130	132	134	135	136	80	80	81	82	83	84	84
	95th	131	132	134	136	138	139	140	84	85	86	87	87	88	89
	99th	139	140	141	143	145	146	147	92	93	93	94	95	96	97

BP, blood pressure

* The 90th percentile is 1.28 SD, 95th percentile is 1.645 SD, and the 99th percentile is 2.326 SD over the mean. For research purposes, the standard deviations in appendix table B–1 allow one to compute BP Z-scores and percentiles for boys with height percentiles given in table 3 (i.e., the 5th, 10th, 25th, 50th, 75th, 90th, and 95th percentiles). These height percentiles must be converted to height Z-scores given by (5% = -1.645; 10% = -1.28; 25% = -0.68; 50% = 0; 75% = 0.68; 90% = 1.28; 95% = 1.645) and then computed according to the methodology in steps 2–4 described in appendix B. For children with height percentiles other than these, follow steps 1–4 as described in appendix B.

Source: The Fourth Report on the Diagnosis, Evaluation, and Treatment of High Blood Pressure in Children and Adolescents, NIH Publication No. 05-5267, http://www.nhlbi.nih.gov/health-pro/guidelines/current/hypertension-pediatric-jnc-4/blood-pressure-tables

Table 1.3

Blood Pressure Levels for Girls by Age and Height Percentile

Age (Year)	BP Percentile ↓	Systolic BP (mmHg) ← Percentile of Height →							Diastolic BP (mmHg) ← Percentile of Height →						
		5th	10th	25th	50th	75th	90th	95th	5th	10th	25th	50th	75th	90th	95th
1	50th	83	84	85	86	88	89	90	38	39	39	40	41	41	42
	90th	97	97	98	100	101	102	103	52	53	53	54	55	55	56
	95th	100	101	102	104	105	106	107	56	57	57	58	59	59	60
	99th	108	108	109	111	112	113	114	64	64	65	65	66	67	67
2	50th	85	85	87	88	89	91	91	43	44	44	45	46	46	47
	90th	98	99	100	101	103	104	105	57	58	58	59	60	61	61
	95th	102	103	104	105	107	108	109	61	62	62	63	64	65	65
	99th	109	110	111	112	114	115	116	69	69	70	70	71	72	72
3	50th	86	87	88	89	91	92	93	47	48	48	49	50	50	51
	90th	100	100	102	103	104	106	106	61	62	62	63	64	64	65
	95th	104	104	105	107	108	109	110	65	66	66	67	68	68	69
	99th	111	111	113	114	115	116	117	73	73	74	74	75	76	76
4	50th	88	88	90	91	92	94	94	50	50	51	52	52	53	54
	90th	101	102	103	104	106	107	108	64	64	65	66	67	67	68
	95th	105	106	107	108	110	111	112	68	68	69	70	71	71	72
	99th	112	113	114	115	117	118	119	76	76	76	77	78	79	79
5	50th	89	90	91	93	94	95	96	52	53	53	54	55	55	56
	90th	103	103	105	106	107	109	109	66	67	67	68	69	69	70
	95th	107	107	108	110	111	112	113	70	71	71	72	73	73	74
	99th	114	114	116	117	118	120	120	78	78	79	79	80	81	81
6	50th	91	92	93	94	96	97	98	54	54	55	56	56	57	58
	90th	104	105	106	108	109	110	111	68	68	69	70	70	71	72
	95th	108	109	110	111	113	114	115	72	72	73	74	74	75	76
	99th	115	116	117	119	120	121	122	80	80	80	81	82	83	83
7	50th	93	93	95	96	97	99	99	55	56	56	57	58	58	59
	90th	106	107	108	109	111	112	113	69	70	70	71	72	72	73
	95th	110	111	112	113	115	116	116	73	74	74	75	76	76	77
	99th	117	118	119	120	122	123	124	81	81	82	82	83	84	84
8	50th	95	95	96	98	99	100	101	57	57	57	58	59	60	60
	90th	108	109	110	111	113	114	114	71	71	71	72	73	74	74
	95th	112	112	114	115	116	118	118	75	75	75	76	77	78	78
	99th	119	120	121	122	123	125	125	82	82	83	83	84	85	86
9	50th	96	97	98	100	101	102	103	58	58	58	59	60	61	61
	90th	110	110	112	113	114	116	116	72	72	72	73	74	75	75
	95th	114	114	115	117	118	119	120	76	76	76	77	78	79	79
	99th	121	121	123	124	125	127	127	83	83	84	84	85	86	87
10	50th	98	99	100	102	103	104	105	59	59	59	60	61	62	62
	90th	112	112	114	115	116	118	118	73	73	73	74	75	76	76
	95th	116	116	117	119	120	121	122	77	77	77	78	79	80	80
	99th	123	123	125	126	127	129	129	84	84	85	86	86	87	88

2   The Fourth Report on the Diagnosis, Evaluation, and Treatment of High Blood Pressure in Children and Adolescents

Continues on next page

Table 1.3 (continued)

Blood Pressure Levels for Girls by Age and Height Percentile

Age (Year)	BP Percentile ↓	Systolic BP (mmHg) ← Percentile of Height →							Diastolic BP (mmHg) ← Percentile of Height →						
		5th	10th	25th	50th	75th	90th	95th	5th	10th	25th	50th	75th	90th	95th
11	50th	100	101	102	103	105	106	107	60	60	60	61	62	63	63
	90th	114	114	116	117	118	119	120	74	74	74	75	76	77	77
	95th	118	118	119	121	122	123	124	78	78	78	79	80	81	81
	99th	125	125	126	128	129	130	131	85	85	86	87	87	88	89
12	50th	102	103	104	105	107	108	109	61	61	61	62	63	64	64
	90th	116	116	117	119	120	121	122	75	75	75	76	77	78	78
	95th	119	120	121	123	124	125	126	79	79	79	80	81	82	82
	99th	127	127	128	130	131	132	133	86	86	87	88	88	89	90
13	50th	104	105	106	107	109	110	110	62	62	62	63	64	65	65
	90th	117	118	119	121	122	123	124	76	76	76	77	78	79	79
	95th	121	122	123	124	126	127	128	80	80	80	81	82	83	83
	99th	128	129	130	132	133	134	135	87	87	88	89	89	90	91
14	50th	106	106	107	109	110	111	112	63	63	63	64	65	66	66
	90th	119	120	121	122	124	125	125	77	77	77	78	79	80	80
	95th	123	123	125	126	127	129	129	81	81	81	82	83	84	84
	99th	130	131	132	133	135	136	136	88	88	89	90	90	91	92
15	50th	107	108	109	110	111	113	113	64	64	64	65	66	67	67
	90th	120	121	122	123	125	126	127	78	78	78	79	80	81	81
	95th	124	125	126	127	129	130	131	82	82	82	83	84	85	85
	99th	131	132	133	134	136	137	138	89	89	90	91	91	92	93
16	50th	108	108	110	111	112	114	114	64	64	65	66	66	67	68
	90th	121	122	123	124	126	127	128	78	78	79	80	81	81	82
	95th	125	126	127	128	130	131	132	82	82	83	84	85	85	86
	99th	132	133	134	135	137	138	139	90	90	90	91	92	93	93
17	50th	108	109	110	111	113	114	115	64	65	65	66	67	67	68
	90th	122	122	123	125	126	127	128	78	79	79	80	81	81	82
	95th	125	126	127	129	130	131	132	82	83	83	84	85	85	86
	99th	133	133	134	136	137	138	139	90	90	91	91	92	93	93

BP, blood pressure

* The 90th percentile is 1.28 SD, 95th percentile is 1.645 SD, and the 99th percentile is 2.326 SD over the mean. For research purposes, the standard deviations in appendix table B–1 allow one to compute BP Z-scores and percentiles for girls with height percentiles given in table 4 (i.e., the 5th, 10th, 25th, 50th, 75th, and 95th percentiles). These height percentiles must be converted to height Z-scores given by (5% = -1.645; 10% = -1.28; 25% = -0.68; 50% = 0; 75% = 0.68; 90% = 1.28; 95% = 1.645) and then computed according to the methodology in steps 2–4 described in appendix B. For children with height percentiles other than these, follow steps 1–4 as described in appendix B.

Source: The Fourth Report on the Diagnosis, Evaluation, and Treatment of High Blood Pressure in Children and Adolescents, NIH Publication No. 05-5267, http://www.nhlbi.nih.gov/health-pro/guidelines/current/hypertension-pediatric-jnc-4/blood-pressure-tables

noncooperative, agitated children are misleading. Attempts must be made to obtain reliable resting measurements. If the child is not quiet, his/her status should be recorded with the blood pressure reading.

    (7) Primary hypertension is detectable in the young, occurring in up to 5 to 10% of children and adolescents.

6. Hypertension is defined as average systolic (SBP) and/or diastolic BP (DBP) that is greater than the 95th percentile for gender, age, and height on more than three occasions.

    a. Prehypertension in children is defined as average SBP or DBP levels that are greater than the 90th percentile but less than the 95th percentile.

    b. As with adults, adolescents with BP levels greater than 120/80 mmHg should be considered prehypertensive.

    c. Elevated BP must be confirmed on repeated visits before characterizing a child as having hypertension.

C. Health history and physical examination vary according to age of the child. Some special considerations for different age groups include the following.

1. 0 to 12 months (infant).

    a. Observe for potential congenital abnormalities or birth injuries.

    b. Assess for growth in terms of length, weight, and head circumference should be made frequently. The most rapid growth rate in life occurs during this time period.

    c. Assess for the development of gross and fine motor skills, language, and social interaction and compare to normal expectations for age. Denver II is a good developmental screening tool and is available in several textbooks.

2. 12 to 36 months (toddler).

    a. Assess growth and development frequently, as for the infant.

    b. Enormous rates of developmental change and a wide range of normal development are observed and require cautious conclusion about delayed development. This is an exploratory stage with many behavioral changes.

    c. Respect parental concern about visual and hearing acuity, eye muscle coordination, and autistic behaviors as these affect the child's long-term adaptive potential.

    d. Provide anticipatory guidance regarding:

        (1) Sleeping patterns.

        (2) Weaning from the bottle.

        (3) Injury prevention.

        (4) Dental hygiene.

        (5) Toilet training and/or regression with illness or sibling birth.

        (6) Separation issues.

3. 4 to 5 years (preschooler).

    a. Survey for normal but slower growth, which continues until puberty.

    b. Formal vision and hearing screening can be tested in this age group.

    c. Identify delays in normal development that might be helped by early childhood intervention programs available in most school systems.

    d. Investigate extremes of uncooperative behaviors toward examiner as these might indicate signs of abnormal development or environmental stresses.

    e. Provide anticipatory guidance regarding:

        (1) Egocentricity.

        (2) Resistance to parental authority; may need to discuss setting limits and consistent discipline.

        (3) Injury prevention.

        (4) Vivid imagination; may need to help differentiate between imagery and lies.

4. 6 to 10 years (school-age).

    a. Begin to elicit aspects of the medical history from the child as well as from the parent or caregiver.

    b. Inquire about participation in activities that can promote physical fitness.

    c. Discuss nutrition, food preferences, and appetite.

    d. Assess dental health and eruption of permanent teeth.

    e. The development of peer groups begins in this age group.

    f. Mood changes and increasing need for privacy emerge.

    g. Provide anticipatory guidance regarding:

        (1) Safety.

        (2) Nutrition.

        (3) Substance abuse.

        (4) Injury prevention.

5. 11 to 12 years (preteen).

    a. Attempt more sophisticated information gathering from the child for history.

    b. Question the patient alone about knowledge of at-risk behaviors, including smoking, alcohol and other substance abuse, and sexual activity.

    c. Provide anticipatory guidance regarding:

        (1) Onset of puberty.

        (2) Changes in body image.

        (3) Peer group interaction.

6. 13 to 18 years (adolescent).

    a. Observe for appearance and maturation of secondary sexual characteristics. Use Tanner stages of development in evaluation of pubertal development (convenient tables with criteria are available at http://www.ncbi.nlm.nih.gov/books/NBK138588/).

b. Observe for pubertal growth spurt. Consider more frequent visits during this time frame to evaluate the effects of kidney disease as the child's growth is rapidly increasing.

c. Obtain history of onset and regularity of menses.

d. Examine for acne, scoliosis, changes in visual acuity, dental caries, and thyromegaly.

e. Question patient alone about at-risk behaviors including sexual activity and smoking, alcohol, and other substance abuse.

f. Address obesity and anorexia issues.

g. Provide anticipatory guidance regarding:
   (1) Sex education.
   (2) Effects of experimentation with alcohol, drugs, cigarettes, etc.
   (3) Hygiene and dental care.
   (4) Nutrition.
   (5) Exercise.
   (6) Safety issues.

D. Physical examination by systems.
   1. General survey.
      a. Alertness, awareness of surroundings, ability to cooperate, evidence of distress.
      b Symmetry, spacing, and position of facial features.
      c. Positioning and posture.
      d. Assessment of size for age and growth curve.
   2. Skin.
      a. Inspect for rashes, especially in the diaper area.
      b. Pigmented, vascular, soft tissue lesions, or skin defects overlying the spine should raise suspicion of an underlying neurologic disorder.
      c. Test tissue turgor and elasticity by gently pinching a fold of abdominal skin and assessing how rapidly it returns to its normal state.
      d. Inspect hands and feet for skin creases and missing or fused digits.
      e. Unusual bruising may be kidney related or signs of abuse.
   3. Head, eyes, ears, nose, and throat (HEENT).
      a. Inspect and palpate head and scalp noting symmetry of shape, bulges or swelling, dilated scalp veins, lesions, lacerations, or protuberances.
      b. Palpate fontanelles, noting early closure or atypical features.
      c. Texture, absence, or abundance of scalp hair may suggest an underlying problem.
      d. Measure frontal occipital circumference (FOC)

until age 3 years and plot on growth grid to assess for trends.

e. Inspect ears for shape, position, and alignment. Perform an exam with an otoscope.

f. Assess hearing. Gross hearing can be assessed by observing infant's or child's physical response to sound. Older children may cooperate with a whisper test.

g. Inspect eyes for size, shape, position, distance between, epicanthal folds, conjunctivae, sclerae (should be white), pupils, swelling, discharge, or excessive tearing.

h. Observe the eyes for tracking. This can also be done in infants.

i. Assess the pupil's response to light, corneal reflex, red reflex. Perform an exam with an ophthalmoscope. Younger children may not cooperate with an exam using an ophthalmoscope. However, after about age 3 to 4 years, they can be taught to cooperate with repetitive examination.

j. Observe teeth for development and dentition.

4. Lymph nodes.
   a. Examination of lymph nodes includes anterior/posterior cervical, occipital, and inguinal nodes. Attention should be given to size, mobility, tenderness, temperature, and condition of overlying skin.
   b. Ages 2 to early adolescent. Superficial, enlarged, freely movable, nontender lymph nodes are easily palpable.
   c. Normally supraclavicular and inguinal nodes are not palpable.

5. Musculoskeletal.
   a. Inspect alignment, symmetry of size, and length of extremities. Observe for unusual masses, protuberances, and joint deformities.
   b. Observe voluntary movements, and flexion. Observe for unusual flacidity or spasticity of extremities.
   c. Examine chest structure, spinal alignment, and structural symmetry. Inspect symmetry of gluteal folds.
   d. Inspect for scoliosis, lumbar lordosis, or thoracic kyphosis.
   e. Palpate bones, muscles, and joints. Assess muscle mass. Palpate to determine areas of tenderness and swelling. Examine hips for evidence of joint dislocation in infants until independently walking.
   f. Observe gait. Note limp or waddle. Observe standing and sitting posture.
   g. The function of joints, range of motion (ROM), bone stability, and muscle strength can be adequately evaluated by observing a child play.

6. Cardiovascular.
   a. Assess chest for symmetry.

b. Palpate chest and precordium. Locate the apical pulse and the point of maximum impulse (PMI). Note any thrills, tap, or heave.

c. Auscultate each cardiac area for S1 and S2, splitting, and murmurs.

   (1) Murmurs in children are frequent and require differentiation between innocent benign murmurs and pathologic murmurs.

   (2) Innocent murmurs are usually soft, short, musical, midsystolic, and heard best in left second and third intercostal spaces.

   (3) Pathologic murmurs may be accompanied by signs of cardiovascular disease (i.e., cyanosis or clubbing).

d. Note the rate and rhythm of the apical pulse. Normal range varies with age. Heart rate in beats per minute (bpm).

   (1) Newborn   120 to 170 bpm.
   (2) 1 year   80 to 160 bpm.
   (3) 3 years   80 to 120 bpm.
   (4) 6 years   75 to 115 bpm.
   (5) 10 years   70 to 110 bpm.

e. Palpate the brachial and radial pulses.

f. Inspect nails for clubbing and assess capillary refill.

g. Palpate inguinal area for femoral pulses.

h. Measure blood pressure (BP).

   (1) Compare to BP standards for age (refer to Tables 1.2 and 1.3 on previous pages).

   (2) Single BP readings are not sufficient to diagnosis hypertension.

   (3) Children with values between the 95th and 99th percentiles are classified as having significant hypertension. When above the 99th percentile, they are considered to have severe hypertension.

7. Pulmonary.

a. Inspect the chest, noting size and shape.

b. Observe the rate, rhythm, and depth of respiration. Note symmetry of chest expansion with respiration.

c. Count the respiratory rate in breaths per minute. The normal range varies with age.

   (1) Newborn   30 to 80 breaths per minute.
   (2) 1 year   20 to 40 breaths per minute.
   (3) 3 years   20 to 40 breaths per minute.
   (4) 6 years   16 to 22 breaths per minute.
   (5) 10 years   16 to 20 breaths per minute.
   (6) 17 years   12 to 20 breaths per minute.

d. Auscultate the breath sounds. Bronchovesicular breath sounds are normally heard because a child's chest is more resonant. Note wheezes, crackles, rubs, prolonged expiration, or prolonged inspiration.

8. Abdomen.

a. Inspect shape, symmetry, configuration, umbilicus, contour, and movement with respiration. Note pulsations or distended veins.

b. Note abdominal protrusion of hernias through umbilicus or rectus abdominis muscle with straining.

c. Auscultate each quadrant for bowel sounds. Bruit or venous hums are abnormal.

d. Palpate lightly and deeply. Note size of liver, spleen, kidney, bladder, masses, or tenderness.

e Percuss each quadrant of the abdomen.

9. Genitourinary.

a. Inspect genitalia.

   (1) Females.

      (a) Inspect labia, clitoris, vaginal introitus, and urethral meatus.

      (b) Determine Tanner pubertal development stage. (Convenient tables with criteria are available in the Adolescent Medicine section of *The Harriett Lane Handbook*, 17th ed.).

   (2) Males.

      (a) Observe penile length, foreskin, location of urethral meatus, scrotal anatomy, presence and location of testes, and presence of abnormal scrotal or inguinal masses.

      (b) Determine Tanner pubertal development stage. (Convenient tables with criteria are available in the Adolescent Medicine section of *The Harriett Lane Handbook*, 17th ed.).

b. Rectum.

   (1) Inspect anal region and perineum for tags, dimples, redness, masses, swelling, or abscesses.

   (2) Digital rectal exam is not usually performed. Deviation from expected stool pattern demands investigation.

10. Neurologic.

a. Neurologic assessment of an older child or adolescent is the same as an adult.

b. Neurologic exam of a younger child or infant.

   (1) Examine on the caregiver's lap, examiner's lap, or bed.

   (2) Observe degree of mental alertness and responsiveness to surroundings in young children.

c. Sensory, motor, and cerebellar examinations require close observation of normal activity, looking for symmetric movement, muscle tone, and strength.

d. Deep tendon reflexes can be elicited at any age.

e. Developmental reflexes present in newborn should disappear within the first year of life: rooting, palmar grasp, Moro, and tonic neck reflexes.

f. Observe head control, position, and movements of the head in first year of life.

g. Evaluate grasp, arm strength, and hand control.
11. Immunization history. Obtain the immunization history and keep up to date. Allergies to medications, foods, and environmental substances should be recorded.

II. Physical findings in kidney failure.

A. General.
1. Uremia may affect wakefulness and mood. The child may be irritable.
2. The presence of kidney disease or other chronic illness may be reflected in failure to thrive.

B. Vital signs.
1. Deviations from normal may be the first indication of CKD.
2. Kidney disease is the most common cause of hypertension in children.
3. Urinary tract infection should be considered when there is an unexplained fever.

C. Growth.
1. Growth retardation, defined as a height below the fifth percentile for age and gender, may result from uremia, metabolic acidosis, osteodystrophy, anemia, or malnutrition associated with kidney failure.
2. Electrolyte and bicarbonate losses should be managed conservatively.
3. Bone abnormalities may result from metabolic acidosis or hyperparathyroidism.
4. Nonresponse to the administration of growth hormone may indicate a need to start kidney replacement therapy (KRT).

D. Skin.
1. Pale, sallow skin may be a sign of kidney-induced anemia.
2. Skin excoriation and infection from scratching may indicate uremia.
3. State of hydration is assessed by examining skin turgor and mucous membranes. Dehydration may be caused by polyuria associated with a child's inability to concentrate urine, causing poor skin turgor and dry mucous membranes.
4. Edema reflects fluid and salt retention.
5. Vasculitic rash, such as the malar butterfly rash of lupus, may indicate an underlying systemic disorder involving the kidneys.
6. Hypopigmented lesions on the trunk and extremities and sebaceous adenomas, similar to acne, appearing between ages 4 and 6 on nose and cheek, are associated with kidney cystic disease.
7. Dysplastic or absent nails may predict kidney disease.

E. HEENT.
1. Preauricular pits and/or deafness frequently occur in association with kidney anomalies such as Alport's syndrome.
2. Watery eyes, photophobia, and cystine crystals throughout the cornea are associated with cystinosis.
3. Cataracts and glaucoma in children are seen in Lowe's syndrome (see Kidney Diseases in Children).

F. Cardiovascular.
1. Kidney disease is the most frequent cause of hypertension in children.
2. Hypervolemia associated with kidney failure may result in tachycardia, gallop rhythm, and hypertension.
3. A heart murmur may reflect a high output state related to anemia.

G. Pulmonary.
1. Dyspnea, coughing, and an increased respiratory rate may indicate fluid overload.
2. Rales and wheezing may also indicate kidney-induced fluid overload.

H. Abdominal.
1. Ascites may be observed in the nephrotic syndrome.
2. Kidney enlargement may cause abdominal distention.
3. Abdominal masses may be caused by hydronephrosis, neoplasms of the kidney, or polycystic kidney disease.

I. Genitourinary.
1. Undescended testes are associated with urinary tract anomalies, such as prune belly syndrome.
2. Absence of a vagina in females is associated with congenital kidney anomalies.
3. History of crying with urination or foul-smelling urine may be signs of urinary tract infection (UTI).
4. Dysuria, urgency, frequency, and hesitancy may or may not be discernible in children.

III. Childhood CKD is staged as in adult CKD.

A. Prior to 2002, children with any level of decreased kidney function were defined as having chronic renal insufficiency.

B. In 2002, with development of the practice guidelines for CKD by the National Kidney Foundation's Kidney Disease Outcomes Quality Initiative (NKF KDOQI), there has been better delineation of the level of kidney disease present.

1. Staging of CKD is essentially the same as for adults. The KDOQI stages of CKD apply to children > 2 years of age (see Table 1.4).
2. For infants eGFR is higher and there is a very wide range of "normal." The following chart should be used for children < 1 year (see Table 1.5).

C. Calculating the estimated glomerular filtration rate (eGFR) is more in-depth in children than in adults due to significant differences in body surface area (BSA).

D. The most accurate and still "gold" standard in measuring the GFR is through iohexol GFR measurement.
   1. Requirements of the test.
      a. Four hours to conduct, making it time consuming.
      b. Two to three separate blood draws.
      c. Injection of iohexol.
   2. There are timed blood draws which reveal the rate of clearance of iohexol and therefore the rate at which the kidneys clear the drug.

E. The most widely used calculation is the Bedside Schwartz Calculation. In children 1 to 18 years of age, eGFR is calculated by using the child's height, serum creatinine (SCr), and a k-constant eGFR = 0.41 x height (cm)/SCr (mg/dl).

F. Cystatin C is becoming more widely used in eGFR calculations.
   1. Cystatin C.
      a. A low molecular weight protein produced by all cells of the body.
      b. It is produced throughout the body at a constant rate and removed and broken down by the kidneys.
      c. It should remain at a steady level in the blood if the kidneys are working efficiently and the GFR is normal.
   2. Cystatin C is postulated to be more closely reflective of the GFR than a serum creatinine alone. Calculations can be done with cystatin C alone, or with creatinine and cystatin C formulas.

IV. Slowing the progression of CKD.

A. Proteinuria.
   1. As in adults, one key to slowing progression of CKD is control of proteinuria.
   2. The type and severity of proteinuria needs to be determined.
      a. Transient proteinuria is a low level of protein excretion (<1 g/24 hours) that can typically follow an illness.
         (1) It is not reproducible for an extended period of time.

Table 1.4

Normal GFR in Neonates, Children, and Adolescents

Age	Mean GFR ± SD (mL/min/1.73 m²)
29–34 weeks GA 1 week postnatal age	15.3 +/−5.6
29–34 weeks GA 2–8 week postnatal age	28.7 +/−13.8
29–34 weeks GA > 8 week postnatal age	51.4
1–week term males and females	41 +/−15
2–8 weeks term males and females	66 +/−25
> 8 weeks term males and females	96 +/−22

GA, Gestational age; *GFR,* glomerular filtration rate; *SD,* standard deviation.

Adapted from Hogget et al. (2003). National Kidney Foundation's Kidney Disease Outcomes Quality Initiative clinical practice guidelines for chronic kidney disease in children and adolescents: Evaluation, classification, and stratification. *Pediatrics, 111*(6),1416-1421.

Table 1.5

Plasma 51Cr-EDTA(creatinine [Cr]-ethylenediaminetetraacetic acid [EDTA]) clearance in normal infants and children

Age (mo)	Mean GFR - SD (mL/min/1.73 m²)
≤ 1.2	52.0 +/−9.0
1.2–3.6	61.7 +/−14.3
3.6–7.9	71.7 +/−13.9
7.9–12	82.6 +/−17.3
12–18	91.5 +/−17.8
18–24	94.5 +/−18.1
> 24	104.4 +/−19.9

Data from Schwartz, G.J., & Work, D.F. (2009). Measurement and estimation of GFR in children and adolescents. *CJASN, 4,*1832-1843.

(2) It usually resolves on its own.
      b. Fixed proteinuria is the presence of elevated protein excretion on > 2 occasions. It is present in morning and evening specimens.
      c. Orthostatic proteinuria is a phenomenon seen most commonly in preadolescents and adolescent patients.
         (1) It is considered a normal variant where protein excretion through the kidney's tubules increases directly in response to amount of time patients are upright.
         (2) It is confirmed with repeat normal values of

morning protein excretion and elevated afternoon/evening specimens.
d. There is also the differentiation between:
  (1) Tubular proteinuria.
    (a) Small protein molecules in the urine; lost from very small capillaries.
    (b) Usually present as a result of scarring.
    (c) Irreversible.
  (2) Glomerular proteinuria.
    (a) Larger protein molecules are present in the urine; lost from renal capillaries.
    (b) This type of proteinuria is amenable to treatment with medications.
3. The main treatment for glomerular fixed proteinuria is an angiotensin converting enzyme inhibitor (ACEi) and/or an angiotensin receptor blocker (ARB).
4. The goal of treatment is to maintain the first morning protein-to-creatinine ratio as close to normal as possible, as blood pressure permits.
5. 24-hour urine collections are impractical in infants and small children; require catheterization.

B. Hypertension.
1. In children, blood pressure goals are based on age, gender, and height percentile as shown in Tables 1.2 and 1.3.
2. Hypertension in children is based on the following parameters.
  a. Hypertension among all adolescents is approximately 3.5%.
  b. Obesity affects approximately 20% of adolescents in the United States, with the incidence of hypertension much higher in the obese (Flynn, 2011).
3. Table 1.6 provides information regarding the treatment of hypertension in children and adolescents.
4. In children with underlying urologic issue(s) or kidney issue(s) including preexisting CKD, the goal is to maintain the blood pressure at or below the 90th percentile for the patient's age and gender.
5. The choice of antihypertensive medication is quite variable unless there is evidence of proteinuria, in which case an angiotensin-converting enzyme inhibitor would be the drug of choice.
6. In 2012, the FDA passed the safety and innovation act (FDASIA). The act encourages funded drug studies to be done in children to better understand the pharmokinetics and safety profiles in children.

C. Lifestyle modification.
1. It is now known that obesity is an independent risk factor for CKD. It has been reported that the risk of CKD stage 5 increases with each unit increase in the body mass index (BMI).
2. Encouraging regular aerobic exercise is paramount.
3. Educate on healthy eating habits including low fat, decreased fried and "fast" foods, modified sodium intake, etc.

V. Areas of focus in childhood CKD based on the stages of CKD.

A. Stage 1 and stage 2 CKD.
1. The primary focus is on prevention as outlined above.
2. The patient may have preexisting issues with electrolyte management based on etiology of the underlying disease processes.

B. Stage 3 CKD.
1. Anemia management.
  a. Iron deficiency.
    (1) Goal: total iron saturation of 20% to 50%.
    (2) Oral iron dosing: 3 to 6 mg/kg/day of elemental iron.
    (3) Intravenous (IV) iron is infrequently used in early stages of CKD. It is considered in cases of significant malabsorption, nonresponsiveness to oral dosing, or severe constipation.
  b. The use of erythropoiesis-stimulating agents (ESAs) is common. Choosing a short- or a long-acting ESA is provider-specific with no long-term benefit of either except less frequent injections.
    (1) Epoetin alfa (Epogen®, Procrit®) dosing is 50 to 150 u/kg given 1 to 3 times a week.
    (2) Darbepoetin alfa (Aranesp®) dosing is either based on a conversion dose from previous epoetin alfa dosing or starting doses of 0.45 mcg/kg/week.
    (3) Response to dosing should be watched carefully.
      (a) A complete blood count (CBC) or hematocrit/hemoglobin (Hct/Hgb) should be checked 2 weeks after starting dose.
      (b) The same holds true after changing a dose.
      (c) Thereafter, a CBC or Hct/Hgb should be drawn monthly for the duration of therapy.
    (4) Side effects of both drugs are similar with the most prevalent being hypertension as a result of a too rapid rise in hemoglobin.
2. Calcium management.
  a. Fluid management is important in calcium management.
  b. Dehydration results in hypercalcemia.
  c. Calcium intake should not be restricted below

Table 1.6

Classification of Hypertension in Children And Adolescents, with Measurement Frequency and Therapy Recommendations

	SBP or DBP Percentile*	Frequency of BP measurement	Therapeutic Lifestyle Changes	Pharmacologic Therapy
Normal	< 90th	Recheck at next scheduled physical examination	Encourage healthy diet, sleep, and physical activity	n/a
Pre-hypertension	90th -< 95th or if BP exceeds 120/80 mm/Hg even if below 90th percentile up to < 95th %ile †	Recheck in 6 months	Weight management counseling if overweight, introduce physical activity and diet management ‡	None unless compelling indications such as CKD, diabetes, heart failure or LVH exist
Stage 1 Hypertension	95th percentile to the 99th percentile + 5mm/Hg	Recheck in 1-2 weeks or sooner if the patient is symptomatic: if persistently elevated on 2 additional occasions, evaluate or refer to source of care within 1 month.	Weight management counseling if overweight, introduce physical activity and diet management.‡	Initiate therapy based on indications
Stage 2 hypertension	> 99th %ile + 5mm/Hg	Evaluate or refer to source of care within 1 week or immediately if patient is symptomatic.	Weight management counseling if overweight, introduce physical activity and diet management ‡	Initiate therapy§

BP = blood pressure; CKD = chronic kidney disease; DBP = diastolic blood pressure; LVH = left ventricular hypertrophy; SBP = systolic blood pressure

* For sex, age, and height measured on at least three separate occasions; if systolic and diastolic categories are different, categorize by the higher value.

† This occurs typically at 12 years old for SBP and at 16 years old for DBP.

‡ Parents and children trying to modify the eating plan to the Dietary Approaches to Stop Hypertension (DASH) eating plan could benefit from consultation with a registered or licensed nutritionist to get them started.

§ More than one drug may be required.

Source: NIH. (2005). *The fourth report on the diagnosis, evaluation, and treatment of high blood pressure in children and adolescents.* http://www.nhlbi.nih.gov/files/docs/resources/heart/hbp_ped.pdf

the daily recommended intake (DRI).

3. Phosphorous management is as difficult in children as it is in adults.
   a. Goals.
      (1) Children birth to 5 years old: 5.5 to 6.5 mg/dL.
      (2) Children over 5 years old: 4.5 to 5. 5 mg/dL.
   b. Dietary restriction of phosphorous is the first-line treatment.
   c. The second focus of therapy is the use of phosphorous (phosphate) binders.
      (1) Calcium-based binders are preferred.
      (2) Children can also use sevelamer.
         (a) Renagel® (sevelamer hydrochloride).
         (b) Renvela® (sevelamer carbonate).
   d. The use of calcimimetics is limited in young children due to concerns with calcium receptors and developing bones.
   e. Lanthanum (Fosrenol®) is not approved in pediatrics.

4. The child's growth can be affected in the earlier stages of CKD when the eGFR is > 70 mL/min/1.73 m². At this point, the effects on growth are probably due to the underlying disease processes coupled with the CKD, rather than solely due to the CKD.
   a. Nutrition is very important and often very complicated in children with CKD from very early on.
   b. A dedicated dietitian is vital to proper maximization of nutritional needs and modification of dietary intake.
   c. As kidney function declines, modifications in protein intake may be necessary.
      (1) This should be kept at the DRI, and not in excessive levels.
      (2) By regulating the protein intake, the kidneys process less protein waste, which reduces waste buildup in the blood.
      (3) It also reduces the workload on the kidneys

and may slow down the progression of kidney disease.

d. Acid base balance is often an issue, especially when urologic abnormalities (e.g., obstructive uropathy) are present.

(1) Supplementation with sodium bicarbonate and sodium chloride is often implemented due to the sodium wasting in polyuric children.

(2) The goal is to have the bicarbonate (CO_2) level maintained at 23 to 30 mEq/L for optimal growth potential.

e. Monitoring weight gain is essential for normal development and brain development.

f. Supplemental nutrition is often necessary.

g. Many children benefit from feeding tubes due to the high volume necessary to maintain their lab values and optimal nutrition.

h. The child's growth in height can be delayed due to the lack of available growth hormone produced by the kidney.

(1) Growth hormone (GH) can be given as a daily injection to supplement growth.

(2) Loss of growth potential is not recoverable, although children will grow "normally" after kidney transplant. Therefore, the use of GH early can prevent overall loss of adult height potential.

(3) Parameters for the initiation of growth hormone include:

(a) Correction of nutritional deficits.

(b) Correction of acidosis – $CO_2 > 22$ mEq/L.

(c) Height percentile < 3rd.

(d) Height standard deviation (SD) score > –2SD.

(e) eGFR < 75 mL/min.

C. Stage 4 CKD.

1. Planning for kidney transplant therapy.

a. Unlike their adult CKD counterparts, in children, preemptive kidney transplant is the treatment plan of choice, therefore avoiding time on dialysis.

b. Transplant evaluation and planning should begin early enough to allow for a preemptive transplant to occur.

2. Kidney replacement therapy (KRT). In some cases, KRT is indicated prior to transplant.

a. Certain immunologic disease processes.

b. Significant social barriers to successful transplantation.

c. Rapid decline in kidney function not allowing for adequate transplant planning time.

D. Stage 5 CKD.

1. Initiation of dialysis.

2. Palliative care planning.

a. A decision may be made to not initiate dialysis when a child is not a transplant candidate or has multiple comorbidities.

b. Palliative dialysis is becoming more widely practiced in pediatrics.

c. Assistance from palliative care teams is preferred.

d. Hospice care will need assistance from the nephrology team to manage CKD comfort issues including uremic urticaria and comfort care medication dosing.

SECTION C
Complications of Kidney Disease in Children

I. Mineral and bone disorders in children with CKD.

A. Children with CKD have potentially long life spans, making optimal control of bone and mineral homeostasis essential for growth, bone health, and cardiovascular health.

B. Kidney Disease Improving Global Outcomes (KDIGO) defines CKD mineral and bone disorder (MBD) as biochemical alterations in the homeostasis of calcium, phosphate, parathyroid hormone (PTH), and vitamin D (Schmitt & Mehis, 2011).

C. Abnormalities in skeletal mineralization occur in a substantial number of children with CKD, including bony deformities and fractures (Wesseling-Perry, 2013).

D. Control of CKD-MBD is essential for prevention of debilitating skeletal complications, growth, and long-term cardiovascular health.

E. Kidney bone disease is impacted by a variety of factors.

1. Acidosis.

2. Calcium and phosphorus imbalance.

3. Elevated levels of parathyroid hormone (PTH).

4. Lack of calcitriol production.

5. Osteocyte dysfunction.

F. Assessment.

1. Left untreated, results in severe kidney osteodystrophy (i.e., rickets).

2. Increased risk for bone fractures and impaired or irregular growth.

G. Nursing care.
   1. Serum phosphorus should be maintained.
      a. Children (ages 1–12) 4.0–6.0 mg/dL (1.45–2.10 mmol/L) (KDOQI, 2006).
      b. Adolescents 3.5–5.5 mg/dL (1.13–1.78 mmol/L).
   2. Administration of phosphate binders.
      a. Phosphate binders should be taken with food, but not with iron supplements.
      b. Phosphate binders enhance excretion of dietary phosphorus.

II. Anemia.

A. Definition and effect on the child (see KDOQI Clinical Practice Recommendations for Pediatrics in Table 1.7).
   1. Anemia contributes to poor quality of life in patients with CKD.
   2. Fatigue, poor cognition, decreased energy, and activity levels.

B. Assessment and diagnosis.
   1. Assess for signs and symptoms of anemia.
      a. Angina, hypotension, tachycardia, and shortness of breath.
      b. Diminished appetite and weight loss.
      c. Decreased sense of well-being.
   2. Review laboratory test results.
      a. Blood urea nitrogen (BUN) and serum creatinine.
      b. Adequacy of dialysis (Kt/Vurea).
      c. CBC.
      d. Iron profile, including serum iron, ferritin, total iron binding capacity (TIBC), and transferrin saturation (TSAT).
   3. Assess for the causes of anemia.
      a. Blood loss.
      b. Iron or vitamin deficiencies.
      c. Inflammation or infection.
      d. Secondary hyperparathyroidism.
      e. Medication interactions.
      f. Coexisting medical conditions.
      g. Malnutrition.
   4. Assess patient and family's understanding of:
      a. The role of kidney in anemia.
      b. Signs and symptoms of anemia.
      c. Consequences of anemia, including left ventricular hypertrophy (LVH).
      d. Signs of gastrointestinal bleeding (e.g., hematemesis, tarry stools).

C. Medical management.
   1. Administer medications needed to treat anemia.
      a. Erythropoiesis-stimulating agents (ESAs).
      b. Iron supplements.
      c. Vitamins.
   2. Monitor response to therapy, including:
      a. Hemoglobin and hematocrit.
      b. Iron profile.
      c. Sense of well-being.
   3. Monitor blood pressure during initiation of therapy with ESAs.

D. Nursing care.
   1. Collaborate with healthcare provider to develop and use an anemia management protocol.
   2. Encourage adherence to treatment and medication routines.
   3. Teach child to self-administer ESA if appropriate to decrease perception of pain.

III. Hypertension.

A. Definition and effect on the child: optimal systolic and diastolic blood pressure should be < 95% for age, gender, and height (refer to Tables 1.2 and 1.3) (NIH, 2004).

B. Assessment and diagnosis.
   1. Hypertension in childhood has become more common as the worldwide obesity rate for children increases (Flynn, 2013).
   2. Data from National Health and Nutrition Examination Survey (NHANES), conducted in the United States between 1999 and 2008, revealed that adolescents 14 to 19 years of age had:
      a. Hypertension in 14% of the participants.
      b. Elevated low-density lipoprotein cholesterol in 22% (Flynn, 2013).

C. Management of BP in children should follow the recommendations of The Fourth Report of the Diagnosis, Evaluation, and Treatment of High Blood Pressure in Children and Adolescents (refer to Table 1.6).

D. Management of hypertension on dialysis requires attention to fluid status, antihypertensive medications, and intradialytic fluid accumulation.
   1. Education by dietitians reinforced regularly.
   2. Limit sodium, usually no more than 2 grams per day.
   3. Increased ultrafiltration (UF) to achieve estimated dry weight (EDW) at each session.
   4. Longer dialysis duration.
   5. More than three dialysis treatments per week or longer sessions.
   6. Antihypertensives for nondialysis days unless child is anephric, then UF alone should be used to control BP.

Table 1.7

KDOQI Clinical Practice Recommendations for Pediatrics

1.1 Identifying Patients and Initiating Evaluation

1.1.1 Stage and cause of CKD: In the opinion of the Work Group, Hb testing should be carried out in all patients with CKD, regardless of stage or cause.

1.1.2 Frequency of testing for anemia: In the opinion of the Work Group, Hb levels should be measured at least annually.

1.1.3 Diagnosis of anemia: PEDIATRIC CPR. In the opinion of the Work Group, in the pediatric patient, diagnosis of anemia should be made and further evaluation should be undertaken whenever the observed Hb concentration is less than the fifth percentile of normal when adjusted for age and sex.

1.2 Evaluation of Anemia in CKD

1.2.1 In the opinion of the Work Group, initial assessment of anemia should include the following tests:

1.2.1.1 CBC including – in addition to the Hb concentration – red blood cell indices (MCH, MCV, MCHC), white blood cell count, and differential and platelet count.

1.2.1.2 Absolute reticulocyte count.

1.2.1.3 Serum ferritin to assess iron stores.

1.2.1.4 PEDIATRIC CPR. In the pediatric patient, serum TSAT to assess adequacy.

2.1 Hb Range

2.1.1 Lower limit of Hb: In patients with CKD, Hb level should be 11.0 g/dL or greater.

2.1.2 Upper limit of Hb: In the opinion of the Work Group, there is insufficient evidence to recommend routinely maintaining Hb levels at 13.0 g/dL or greater in ESA-treated patients.

CPR For Pediatric 3.1 Using ESAs

3.1.1 Frequency of Hb monitoring.

3.1.1.1 In the opinion of the Work Group, frequency of Hb monitoring in patients treated with ESAs should be at least monthly.

3.1.2 ESA dosing:

3.1.2.1 In the opinion of the Work Group, the initial ESA dose and ESA dose adjustments should be determined by the patient's Hb level, the target Hb level, the observed rate of increase in the Hb level, and clinical circumstances.

3.1.2.2 In the opinion of the Work Group, ESA doses should be decreased, but not necessarily held, when a downward adjustment of Hb level is needed.

3.1.2.3 In the opinion of the Work Group, scheduled ESA doses that have been missed should be replaced at the earliest possible opportunity.

3.1.2.4 In the opinion of the Work Group, ESA administration in ESA-dependent patients should continue during hospitalization.

3.1.2.5 In the opinion of the Work Group, hypertension, vascular access occlusion, inadequate dialysis, histories of seizures, or compromised nutritional status are not contraindications to ESA therapy.

3.1.3 Route of administration:

3.1.3.1 PEDIATRIC CPR. In the opinion of the Work Group, in the pediatric patient, the route of administration should be determined by the CKD stage, treatment setting, efficacy considerations, the class of ESA used, and the anticipated frequency and pain of administration.

3.1.3.2 In the opinion of the Work Group, convenience favors SC administration in non-HD-CKD patients.

3.1.3.3 In the opinion of the Work Group, convenience favors IV administration in patients with HD-CKD.

3.1.4 Frequency of administration:

3.1.4.1 PEDIATRIC CPR. In the opinion of the Work Group, in the pediatric patient, the frequency of administration should be determined by the CKD stage, treatment setting, efficacy consideration, and the class of ESA; as well, consideration should be given to the anticipated frequency of, and pain on administration of, each agent and their potential effects on the child and family.

3.1.4.2 In the opinion of the Work Group, convenience favors less frequent administration, particularly in non-HD-CKD patients.

CPR for Pediatrics 3.2 Using iron agents

3.2.1 Frequency of iron status tests: In the opinion of the Work Group, iron status tests should be performed as follows:

3.2.1.1 Every month during initial ESA treatment.

3.2.1.2 At least every 3 months during stable ESA treatment or in patients with HD-CKD not treated with ESA.

3.2.2 Interpretation of iron status tests: In the opinion of the Work Group, results of iron status tests, HB level, and ESA dose should be interpreted together to guide iron therapy.

3.2.3 Targets of iron therapy: In the opinion of the Work Group, sufficient iron should be administrated to generally maintain the following indices of iron status during ESA treatment:

3.2.3.1 PEDIATRIC CPR HD-CKD:
- Serum ferritin > 100 ng/mL; AND
- TSAT > 20%.

3.2.3.2 ND-CKD and PKD-CKD:
- Serum ferritin > 100 ng/mL AND
- TSAT > 20%.

3.2.4 Upper level of ferritin: In the opinion of the Work Group, there is insufficient evidence to recommend routine administration of IV iron if serum ferritin is greater than 500 ng/mL. When ferritin level is greater than 500 ng/mL, decisions regarding IV iron administration should weigh ESA responsiveness, Hb and TSAT level, and the patient's clinical status.

Continues on next page

Table 1.7 (page 2 of 4) ———— KDOQI Clinical Practice Recommendations for Pediatrics

3.2.5 Route of administration:

3.2.5.1 The preferred route of administration is IV in patients with HD-CKD.

3.2.5.2 In the opinion of the Work Group, the route of iron administration can be either IV or oral in patients with ND-CKD and PD-CKD.

3.2.6 Hypersensitivity reactions: In the opinion of the Work Group, resuscitative medication and personnel trained to evaluate the resuscitate anaphylaxis should be available whenever a dose of iron dextran is administered.

CPR For Pediatrics 3.3 Using Pharmacological and Nonpharmacological Adjuvants to ESA Treatment in HD-CKD

3.3.1 L-carnitine: (FULLY APPLICABLE TO CHILDREN) In the opinion of the Work Group, there is sufficient evidence to recommend the use of L-carnitine in the management of anemia in patients with CKD.

3.3.2 Vitamin C: (FULLY APPLICABLE TO CHILDREN) In the opinion of the Work Group, there is insufficient evidence to recommend the use of vitamin C (ascorbate) in the management of anemia in patients with CKD.

3.3.3 Androgens: (FULLY APPLICABLE TO CHILDREN) Androgens should not be used as an adjuvant to ESA treatment in anemic patients with CKD. (STRONG RECOMMENDATION)

Clinical Practice Guideline 6. Pediatric Peritoneal Dialysis

6.1 Recommended laboratory measurements for peritoneal membrane function:

6.1.1 The PET is the preferred approach to the clinical assessment of peritoneal membrane transport capacity in pediatric patients and should be performed to aid in the prescription process. (A)

6.2 Maintenance of euvolemia and normontension:

6.2.1 The frequent presence of hypertension and associated cardiac abnormalities in children receiving PD requires strict management of blood pressure, including attention to fluid status. (A)

6.3 Quality improvement programs:

6.3.1 The CQI process has shown to improve outcomes in many disciplines, including CKD stage 5. (A)

6.3.1.1 Each home training unit should establish quality improvement programs with the goal of monitoring clinical outcomes and implementing programs that result in improvements in patient care. In children, growth and school attendance/performance are clinical activities to be monitored in addition to those recommended for adult patients.

6.3.1.2 Quality improvement programs should include representatives of all disciplines involved in the care of pediatric PD patient, including physicians, nurses, social workers, dietitians, play therapists, psychologists, and teachers.

6.3.1.3 Single-center trends in pediatric clinical outcomes should be compared with national and international data.

Clinical Practice Recommendations for Guideline 6: Pediatric Peritoneal Dialysis

6.1 Dialysis initiation:

6.1.1 Dialysis initiation should be considered for the pediatric patient

6.2 Modality selection:

6.2.1 The decision regarding the selection of PD as a dialysis modality for the pediatric patient should take a variety of factors into account, including patient/family choice, patient size, medical comorbidities, and family support.

6.3 Quality improvement programs:

6.3.1 The CQI process has been shown to improve outcomes in many disciplines, including CKD stage 5. (A)

6.3.1.1 Each home training unit should establish quality improvement programs with the goal of monitoring clinical outcomes and implementing programs that result in improvements in patient care. In children, growth and school attendance/performance are clinical activities to be monitored in addition to those recommended for adult patients.

6.3.1.2 Quality improvement programs should include representatives of all disciplines involved in the care of the pediatric PD patient, including physicians, nurses, social workers, dietitians, play therapists, psychologists, and teachers.

6.3.1.3 Single-center trends in pediatric clinical outcomes should be compared with national and international data.

6.3 **Solute clearance targets and measurements:**

6.3.1 In the absence of definitive data correlating solute removal and clinical outcome in children, current recommendations for solute clearance in pediatric patients receiving PD are as follows:

6.3.1.1 The pediatric patient's clinical status should be reviewed at least monthly, and delivery of the prescribed solute clearance should render the patient free of signs and symptoms of uremia.

6.3.1.2 All measurements of peritoneal solute clearance should be obtained when the patient is clinically stable and at least 1 month after resolution of an episode of peritonitis.

6.3.1.3 More frequent measurements of peritoneal solute clearance and RKF should be considered when clinical events are likely to have resulted in decreased clearance or when new/worsening signs or symptoms of uremia develop.

6.3.1.4 Regardless of the delivered dose of dialysis, if a patient is not doing well and has no other identifiable cause other than kidney failure, a trial of increased dialysis is indicated.

6.3.2 For patients with RKF (defined as urine $Kt/V_{urea} > 0.1/wk$):

Continues on next page

Table 1.7 (page 3 of 4) ———— **KDOQI Clinical Practice Recommendations for Pediatrics**

6.3.2.1 The minimal "delivered" dose of total (peritoneal and kidney) small-solute clearance should be a Kt/V$_{urea}$ of at least 1.8/wk.

6.3.2.2 Total solute clearance should be a measured within the first month after initiating dialysis and at least once every 6 months thereafter.

6.3.2.3 If the patient has FKF and residual kidney clearance is being considered as part of the patient's total weekly solute clearance, determinations should be obtained at a minimum of every 3 months.

6.3.3 For patients with RKF (defined as urine Kt/V$_{urea}$ < 0.1/wk) or for those in whom RKF is unable to be measured accurately:

6.3.3.1 The minimal "delivered" dose of small-solute clearance determinations should be a peritoneal Kt/V$_{urea}$ of at least 1.8/wk.

6.3.3.2 The peritoneal solute clearance should be measured within the first month after starting dialysis and at least once every 6 months thereafter.

6.3.4 When calculating Kt/V$_{urea}$, one should estimate V or TBW by using the sex-specific nomograms based upon the following equations:
Males: TBW = 0.010 · (height · weight)$^{0.68}$ − 0.37 · weight
Females: TBW = 0.14 · (height · weight)$^{0.64}$ − 0.35 · weight

Reprinted with permission from National Kidney Foundation 2006 Updates

6.4 **Preservation of RKF:**

6.4.1 Techniques that may contribute to the preservation of RKF in pediatric patients receiving PD should be incorporated as a component of dialysis care whenever possible.

6.4.1.1 Nephrotoxic insults in those with normal or impaired kidney function should be assumed, in the absence of direct evidence, to also be nephrotoxic in patients on PD therapy who have RFK and therefore should be avoided.

6.4.1.2 Aminoglycoside antibiotics should be avoided whenever possible to minimize the risk for nephrotoxicity, as well as ototoxicity and vestibular toxicity.

6.4.1.3 "Prekidney" and "postkidney" causes of a decrease in RKF should be considered in the appropriate clinical setting.

6.4.1.4 Infections of the urinary tract should be treated promptly.

6.4.1.5 Diuretics should be used to maximize urinary salt and water excretion.

6.4.1.6 An ACE inhibitor or ARB should be considered in a PD patient who requires antihypertensive medication and had RKF.

Reprinted with permission from National Kidney Foundation 2006 Updates

6.5 **Writing the PD prescription:**

6.5.1 In addition to solute clearance, QOL, ultrafiltration/volume control, and possibly the clearance of middle molecules should be considered when writing the PD prescription.

6.5.1.1 The patient's dialysis schedule and QOL, as it relates to such issues as school and work attendance/performance, should be taken into account when designing the dialysis prescription.

6.5.1.2 To optimize small-solute clearance, minimize cost, and possibly decrease the frequency of exchanges, one should first increase the instilled volume per exchange (target range, 1,000 to 1,200 mL/m^2 BSA; maximum, 1,400 mL/m^2 BSA), as tolerated by the patient, before increasing the number of exchanges per day. The volume of the supine exchange(s) should be increased first because this position has the lowest intraabdominal pressure. Objective evidence of patient tolerance may require assessment of IPP.

6.5.1.3 The patient's record of PD effluent volume from the overnight dwell of CAPD and daytime dwell of CCPD.

6.5.1.4 Factors to be considered when attempting to optimize total body volume include:
a. Dietary sodium and fluid restriction may be implemented in patients unable to maintain euvolemia/normotension with dialysis alone.
b. In patients with RKF, diuretics may be preferred over increasing the dialysate dextrose concentration to achieve euvolemia.
c. Drain volume should be optimized after the overnight dwell of CAPD and the daytime dwell(s) of CCPD to maximize solute clearance and ultrafiltration volume.
d. In patients who are hypertensive or in whom there is evidence of volume overload, ultrafiltration generally should be positive for all daytime or nighttime exchanges.
e. An effort should be made to determine the lowest possible dialysate dextrose concentration required to achieve the desired ultrafiltration volume.

6.5.1.5 To optimize middle-molecule clearance in patients who have minimal RKF, the PD prescription should preferentially include the use of CCPD with dwells 24 hr/day or CAPD. This is recommended even if small-molecule clearance is above target without the longer dwell.

6.5.1.6 The use of NIPD (e.g., no daytime dwell) can be considered in pediatric patients who are clinically well, whose combined dialysis prescription and RKF achieves or exceeds the target solute clearance, and who are without evidence of hyperphosphatemia, hyperkalemia, hypervolemia, or acidosis.

Reprinted with permission from National Kidney Foundation 2006 Updates

6.6 **Other aspects of the care of the pediatric PD patient:**

6.6.1 All children on PD therapy with anemia should follow the KDOQI Guidelines for Management of Anemia that pertain to pediatrics.

6.6.2 Management of dyslipidemias for prepubertal children on PD therapy should follow recommendations by the National Cholesterol Expert Panel in Children and Adolescents. Postpubertal children or adolescents on

Continues on next page

Table 1.7 (page 4 of 4) ———KDOQI Clinical Practice Recommendations for Pediatrics

PD therapy should follow the pediatric recommendations provided in the KDOQI Clinical Practice Guidelines for Managing Dyslipidemia in CKD.

6.6.3   All children on PD therapy should follow the pediatric-specific recommendations provided in the KDOQI Clinical Practice Guidelines on Hypertension and Antihypertensive Agents in CKD.

6.6.4   All children on PD therapy should follow the recommendations provided in the KDOQI Clinical Practice Guidelines for Nutrition in Chronic Renal Failure.

Reprinted with permission from National Kidney Foundation 2006 Updates

Clinical Practice Guideline 8.
Pediatric Hemodialysis Prescription and Adequacy

8.1   Initiation of HD:

8.1.1   Dialysis initiation considerations for the pediatric patient should follow the adult patient guideline of a GFR less than 15 mL/ min/1.73 m^2. (A)

8.1.2   For pediatric patients, GFR can be estimated by using either a timed urine collectionor the Schwartz formula. (A)

8.1.3   Dialysis therapy initiation should be considered at higher estimated GFRs when the patient's clinical course is complicated by the presence of the signs and symptoms listed in Table 15.5, CPR 1 for adult patients, as well as malnutrition or growth failure for pediatric patients. Before dialysis is undertaken, these conditions should be shown to be refractory to medications and/or dietary management. (A)

Reprinted with permission from National Kidney Foundation 2006 Updates

Clinical Practice Recommendation 8:
Vascular Access in Pediatric Patients

8.1   Choice of access type:

8.1.1   Permanent access in the form of a fistula or graft is the preferred form of vascular access for most pediatric patients on maintenance HD therapy.

8.1.2   Circumstances in which a CVC may be acceptable for pediatric long-term access include lack of local surgical expertise to place permanent vascular access in small children, patient size too small to support a permanent vascular access, bridging HD for PD training or PD catheter removal for peritonitis, and expectation of expeditious kidney transplantation.

8.1.3   If surgical expertise to place permanent access does not exist in the patient's pediatric setting, efforts should be made to consult vascular access expertise among local adult-oriented surgeons to either supervise or place permanent vascular access in children.

8.1.4   Programs should evaluate their patients' expected waiting times on their local decreased-donor kidney transplant waiting lists. Serious consideration should be given to placing permanent vascular access in children greater than 20 kg in size who are expected to wait more than 1 year for a kidney transplant.

8.2   Stenosis surveillance: An AVG stenosis surveillance protocol should be established to detect venous anastomosis stenosis and direct patients for surgical revision or PTA.

8.3   Catheter sizes, anatomic sites, and configurations:

8.3.1   Catheter sizes should be matched to patient sizes with the goal of minimizing intraluminal trauma and obstruction to blood flow while allowing sufficient blood flow for adequate HD.

8.3.2   External cuffed access should be placed in the internal jugular with the distal tip placed in the right atrium.

8.3.3   The BFR of an external access should be minimally 3 to 5 mL/kg/min and should be adequate to deliver the prescribed HD dose.

8.2   Measurement of HD adequacy:

8.2.1   spKt, calculated by either formula urea kinetic modeling or the second-generation natural logarithm formula, should be used for month-to-month assessment of delivered HD dose. (B)

8.2.2   Assessment of nutrition status as an essential component of HD adequacy measurement. nPCR should be measured monthly by using either formula urea kinetic modeling or algebraic approximation. (B)

8.2.3   Principles and statements regarding slow-flow methods for postdialysis sampling and inclusion of RKF (or lack thereof) outlined in the adult guideline also pertain to pediatric patients. (B)

8.3   Prescription of adequate HD:

8.3.1   Children should receive at least the delivered dialysis dose as recommended for the adult population. (A)

8.3.2   For younger pediatric patients, prescription of higher dialysis dose and higher protein intakes at 150% of the recommended nutrient intake for age may be important. (B)

8.4   Non-dose-related components of adequacy:
Accurate assessment of patient intravascular volume during the HD treatment should be provided to optimize ultrafiltration. (B)

Reprinted with permission from National Kidney Foundation 2006 Updates

E. Patients on dialysis should have pulse pressure (PP) determined monthly before dialysis (see section on fluid removal in pediatric hemodialysis). When the PP is greater than 60 mmHg and systolic BP greater than 135 mmHg:
 1. Reduce by achieving ideal body weight and using antihypertensive medication.
 2. Continue efforts until able to reach EDW and a target PP of 40 mmHg.

IV. Cardiovascular disease (CVD).

A. Definition and effect on the child.
 1. Causes of deaths due to cardiovascular events (USRDS, 2013).
  a. Cardiac arrest (cause uncertain) in 25%.
  b. Stroke 16%.
  c. Myocardial ischemia 14%.
  d. Pulmonary edema 12%.
  e. Hyperkalemia 11%.
  f. Other cardiovascular causes, including arrhythmia in 22%.
 2. Cardiovascular disease was the leading cause of death in pediatric patients on dialysis in 2013 USRDS data.
 3. Cardiac complications, such as congestive heart failure and arrhythmias, are of particular concern in pediatric patients for whom fluid overload and hypertension are major clinical problems (USRDS, 2013).
  a. Arrhythmias include sinus tachycardia, premature ventricular contractions (PVC), and heart block in pediatric patients on chronic dialysis.
  b. Atherosclerosis (AHD) is prevalent in 10 to 15% of pediatric chronic patients on dialysis (more common when the serum phosphorus and the calcium-phosphorus product are elevated).
  c. Coronary artery calcification was associated with higher levels of C-reactive protein (CRP), plasma homocysteine, intact PTH, and higher calcium-phosphorus product.
 4. Echocardiography should be used to document left ventricular hypertrophy (LVH), left ventricular dilation, and cardiomyopathy (systolic and diastolic dysfunction):
  a. When the patient begins dialysis.
  b. Once the patient has achieved dry weight.
  c. Then at 3-year intervals.
 5. LVH is a known risk factor for CVD and mortality in adults on chronic dialysis and may well also contribute to CVD risk in children.
 6. Valvular heart disease (VHD) should be evaluated by echocardiography.

B. Assessment and diagnosis. KDOQI guidelines recommend children starting dialysis be evaluated for the presence of cardiac disease (i.e., cardiomyopathy and valvular disease).
 1. Echocardiogram once patient achieves dry weight (ideally within 3 months).
 2. Screen for dyslipidemias.
 3. Screen for hypertension.

C. Medical management.
 1. VHD should be managed following ACC/AHA guidelines.
 2. When dialysis is initiated, patients should have a 12-lead electrocardiogram (ECG). It should be repeated once the dry weight is achieved, ideally within 3 months.
 3. Screen for traditional CVD risk factors, such as dyslipidemia and hypertension.
 4. Strict adherence to achieving the EDW and controlling the BP at each dialysis session, especially in the anephric patient.
 5. Intact PTH assay (first-generation immunoradiometric assay) should be monitored every 3 months. The targeted goal for the prevention of CVD is between 150 and 300 pg/mL (16.5 to 33.0 pmol/L).

D. Nursing care.
 1. Onsite automatic external defibrillator (AED) and/or appropriate pediatric equipment should be kept available and in good working order.
 2. Use pediatric arrhythmia algorithm.
 3. Basic life support (BLS) and pediatric advanced life support (PALS) are important.

V. Infection.

A. Definition and effect on the child.
 1. Infection is the second largest cause of death in pediatric patients on chronic dialysis, accounting for 20% of deaths in that patient population (USRDS, 2013).
 2. More children have central venous catheters than in the adult population.
 3. Infections can lead to poor performance in school due to lost school days.
 4. Rates of infectious hospitalization constitute almost half of the admissions per year (USRDS, 2013).
 5. Infections are now tracked by the CDC via NHSN.

B. Assessment and diagnosis.
 1. Monitor for temperature elevations.
 2. Monitor C-reactive protein (CRP) for inflammation.
 3. Evaluate and treat suspected infections. Children with lines in place can develop chronic line infections.

C. Medical management.
1. Obtain cultures and administer antibiotics. Adjust treatment based on results of culture and sensitivity reports.
2. Evaluate for methicillin-resistant staph (MRSA).

D. Nursing care.
1. Careful questioning to ascertain possible source of infection.
2. Patient and family education is a vital part of any pediatric dialysis program.

SECTION D
Acute Kidney Injury

I. Definition.

A. Acute kidney injury (AKI) is an abrupt decrease in kidney function encompassing various etiologies.

B. AKI encompasses previous terms, acute kidney failure (AKF), acute renal failure (ARF), or acute tubular necrosis (ATN).

C. AKI is defined as any one of the following (KDIGO, 2012a).
1. Increase in serum creatinine by 0.3 mg/dL within 48 hours.
2. Increase in serum creatinine to 1.5 times baseline level.
3. Urine volume 0.5 ml/kg/h for 6 hours.

D. AKI is associated with increased hospital length of stay, mortality, and morbidity.

II. AKI Staging and/or Classification.

A. AKI staging or classification is based on the severity of the injury.
1. Several different classifications or stagings have been proposed, including RIFLE, pediatric RIFLE (pRIFLE), and AKIN systems.
2. Yet, since a single definition was needed, KDIGO proposed a staging system that incorporates RIFLE, pRIFLE, and AKIN classifications: AKI staging (KDIGO, 2012a).

B. AKI Staging by Kidney Disease Improving Global Outcomes (KDIGO) is shown in Table 1.8.

III. Common causes of acute kidney injury.

A. Prerenal injury results from decreased perfusion to the kidney.

Table 1.8

Staging of AKI

STAGE	SERUM CREATININE	URINE OUTPUT
1	1.5–1.9 baseline OR ≥ 0.3 mg/dL (≥ 26.5µmol/l increase	< 0.5mL/kg/h for 6–12 hours
2	2.0–2.9 times baseline	< 0.5 mL/kg/h for ≥ 12 hours
3	3.0 baseline OR Increase in creatinine to ≥ 4.0 mg/dL (≥ 353.6 µmol/l) OR Initiation of renal replacement therapy OR In patients < 18 years, decrease in eGFR to < 135 mL/min per 1.73 m^2	< 0.3 mL/kg/h for ≥ 24 hours OR Anuria for ≥ 12 hours

Used with permission from KDIGO (2012). *Clinical practice guideline for acute kidney injury.* Retrieved from http://kdigo.org/home/guidelines/acute-kidney-injury

1. Volume depletion (bleeding, intestinal losses, burns).
2. Decreased cardiac output (heart failure).
3. Liver failure (hepatorenal syndrome).
4. Hypoalbuminemic states (nephrotic syndrome, sepsis).

B. Structural kidney injury (previously termed intrinsic kidney injury or acute tubular necrosis) results from structural damage to the kidney vasculature, glomeruli, or tubules.
1. Hypoxia/ischemic insult.
2. Nephrotoxic medication exposure.
   a. Antibiotics – aminoglycosides, penicillins, vancomycin, pipercillin, cephalosporins, sulfonamides, rifampin, ciprofloxacin, tetracyclines.
   b. Nonsteroidal anti-inflammatory drugs – ibuprofen, naprosyn, ketorolac.
   c. COX-2 inhibitors.
   d. Contrast agents.
   e. Chemotherapeutic agents – methotrexate, cisplatin, ifosfamide.
   f. Others – acyclovir.
3. Rhabdomyolysis.
4. Tumor lysis syndrome.
5. Ethylene glycol toxicity.
6. Hemolytic uremic syndrome.
7. Thrombosis (renal vein or renal artery).
8. Poststreptococcal glomerulonephritis or postinfectious glomerulonephritis.

C. Postkidney injury results from bilateral urinary tract obstruction.
   1. Renal calculi.
   2. Uncorrected congenital obstructive uropathies.
   3. Urethral obstructions.

IV. Neonatal (very low birth weight) considerations.

A. Diagnosing AKI is difficult because very low birth weight (VLBW) infants start with a low GFR which varies greatly depending on the degree of prematurity (Askenazi et al., 2009).

B. Serum creatinine in the first few days of life reflects the mother's rather than the infant's kidney function.

C. Small changes in the creatinine reflect significant changes in kidney function.

D. Neonatal specific causes of AKI.
   1. Low birth APGAR scores.
   2. Severe asphyxia at birth.
   3. Maternal ingestion of antibiotics or NSAIDs.

V. Kidney replacement therapy for AKI.

A. Hemodialysis (HD): pediatric and neonatal considerations with HD.
   1. The patient's size is a unique challenge: filters and tubing sets may be too large in comparison to patient size.
   2. Priming the circuit with blood should be considered for any patient for which the circuit's volume is > 10% of the patient's estimated blood volume (Bunchman et al., 2008).
   3. Fluid removal using noninvasive blood volume monitoring is recommended to optimize ultrafiltration. Noninvasive blood volume monitoring reduces intradialytic symptoms such as hypotension, nausea, vomiting, cramping, and headaches (Michael et al., 2004).

B. Peritoneal dialysis (PD): pediatric and neonatal considerations with PD.
   1. The catheter can be placed in the operating room or a temporary catheter can be placed at the bedside in critical care units.
   2. Smaller catheters are necessary for the neonate or infant.
   3. Initial fill volumes are 10 mL/kg.
   4. Manual dialysis exchanges may be necessary for volumes less than 100 mL.
   5. Manual dialysis is time intensive, requiring constant monitoring to perform the fill and drain procedures.
   6. Neonates and infant fluid removal may be very

sensitive to the dextrose-containing peritoneal solutions.

C. Continuous renal replacement therapy (CRRT).
   1. Indications for CRRT.
      a. Fluid management.
         (1) Fluid overload. An increase in positive fluid accumulation of 10% of body weight is associated with increased mortality and morbidity (Sutherland et al., 2010).
         (2) Hemodynamic instability on intermittent hemodialysis.
         (3) Provide adequate nutritional support.
      b. Solute management.
         (1) Correct electrolyte imbalances.
         (2) Correct metabolic disturbances: inborn errors of metabolism, trauma, other acid/base imbalances.
   2. Advantages of CRRT.
      a. Minimization of hypotensive episodes.
      b. Provision of continuous solute clearances.
      c. Provision of continuous toxin removal.
      d. Minimization of the shifts in intracranial pressure due to rapid chemical clearances associated with dialysis disequilibrium.
      e. CRRT machines are safe with accurate fluid infusions and removal.
      f. May promote kidney function recovery compared to HD.
   3. Pediatric and neonatal considerations with CRRT.
      a. Patient size is a unique challenge: filters and tubing sets may be too large in comparison to patient size (Bunchman et al., 2008; Michael et al., 2004).
      b. Priming the circuit with blood should be considered for any patient that the circuit volume is > 10% of the estimated patient's blood volume.
      c. The use of AN-69 membranes requires special techniques to avoid bradykinin release syndrome when priming the circuit with blood (Brophy et al., 2001).
      d. Vascular access is a challenge for this patient population (Hackbarth et al., 2007).
         (1) Sites for the catheter include femoral, internal jugular, or subclavian. The subclavian is the least preferred site due to potential for subclavian venous stenosis.
         (2) Double lumen catheters are preferred, but two single lumen catheters can be used.
   4. Nursing considerations with CRRT.
      a. Careful continuous monitoring for complications is required for:
         (1) Hypotension.
         (2) Excessive fluid removal.
         (3) Electrolyte and acid-base imbalances.
         (4) Hypothermia. Blood warmers may not be

adequate for maintaining normal temperature. Other external warming measures may be necessary.

(5) Bleeding.

(6) Infections.

(7) Blood leaks from the filter.

(8) Clotting filter or circuit.

(9) Inadequate blood flow through the catheter and the circuit.

b. Vascular access problems will limit the effectiveness of the therapy if not resolved.

c. The child should never be left alone while on the treatment.

VI. Outcomes.

A. Short-term outcomes.

1. Children with AKI requiring kidney replacement therapy have a survival rate, defined as discharge from the intensive care unit, of approximately 50 to 60% (Symons et al., 2007).

2. Infants with AKI requiring KRT have a survival rate, defined as discharge from the intensive care unit, of 35 to 44% (Askenazi et al., 2013).

B. Long-term outcomes: 45–50% of children with an AKI episode have one sign of chronic kidney disease 3 to 5 years after the episode. This could include:

1. Hyperfiltration.

2. Reduced kidney function.

3. Hypertension.

4. Microalbuminuria (Askenazi et al., 2006; Mammen et al., 2012).

Section E
Kidney Replacement Therapies

Patients with an estimated glomerular filtration rate < 30 mL/min/1.73 m² (CKD stage 4) should be educated on all modalities of kidney replacement therapy options: PD, home HD, in-center HD, transplantation, and palliative care. Timely referrals allow for placement of a permanent dialysis access if necessary.

I. Pediatric kidney transplantation.

A. Preferred mode of therapy for pediatric patients with CKD stage 5 (Sayed et al., 2013).

B. Contraindications for transplantation in children.

1. Absolute and serious contraindications. (*Note:* These may vary slightly from center to center.)

a. Active or untreated malignancy.

b. Chronic HIV infection.

c. Chronic active infection with hepatitis B.

d. Severe multiorgan failure.

e. Positive current direct crossmatch.

f. Debilitating irreversible brain injury.

g. Size < 10 kg.

h. Anatomy incompatible with transplant procedure, such as no available blood vessels.

i. Unable to tolerate the surgical procedure, such as severe pulmonary compromise or severe bleeding.

2. Relative contraindications.

a. Coronary or pulmonary disease that places the patient at high risk.

b. HIV infection.

c. Sickle cell disease.

d. Active chronic systemic illness that requires maintenance corticosteroid therapy (e.g., lupus).

e. Urinary issues.

f. Severe malnutrition.

g. Severe obesity (BMI > 38 kg/m²).

h. Active infection.

i. Risk of recurrence of initial disease.

j. Significant cognitive deficit without reliable caregiver.

k. Active illegal drug use.

l. Ongoing nonadherence.

m. Resources deemed inadequate for follow-up care.

C. The pretransplant evaluation/preparation. *Note:* The etiology of the kidney failure can directly impact when a child may be transplanted.

1. Causes of kidney failure.

a. Aplasia/hypoplasia/dysplasia kidney.

b. Obstructive uropathy.

c. Focal segmental glomerulosclerosis/ glomerulonephritis/nephritis.

d. Reflux nephropathy.

e. Polycystic disease/medullary cystic disease.

f. Congenital nephrotic syndrome.

g. Hemolytic uremic syndrome.

h. Prune belly.

i Cystinosis.

j. Systemic lupus erythematosus (SLE) nephritis.

k. Renal infarct.

l. Berger's (IgA) nephritis.

m. Henoch-Schonlein nephritis.

n. Wegener's granulomatosis.

o. Wilm's tumor.

p. Drash syndrome.

q. Oxalosis.

r. Membranous nephropathy.

s. Other systemic immunologic diseases.

t. Other (NAPRTCS, 2010).

2. Frequency of transplantation: From 2009 to 2011,

2371 pediatric (under age 17) patients received a kidney transplant (OPTN, 2011).

  3. Donor source.

    a. Living donor (LRD vs LURD).

      (1) Parent: 40.2% (NAPRTCS, 2012).

      (2) Other living donor: 10.5% (NAPRTCS, 2012).

    b. Deceased donor: 49.2% (NAPRTCS, 2012).

      (1) Brain death.

        (a) Irreversible cessation of cerebral and brain stem function; characterized by absence of electrical activity in the brain, blood flow to the brain, and brain function as determined by clinical assessment of responses.

        (b) A brain dead person is dead, although his or her cardiopulmonary functioning may be artificially maintained for some time (UNOS glossary).

      (2) Non-heart-beating: recovery of organs and/or tissues from a donor whose heart has irreversibly stopped beating, previously referred to as non-heart-beating or asystolic donation (UNOS).

      (3) Expanded criteria: a kidney donated for transplantation from any brain dead donor over the age of 60 years, or from a donor over the age of 50 years with two of the following:

        (a) A history of hypertension.

        (b) The most recent serum creatinine greater than or equal to 1.5 mg/dL.

        (c) Death resulting from a cerebral vascular accident (stroke) (UNOS).

    c. Altruistic donor.

      (1) This is a person who comes forward to donate to another person.

      (2) They offer to donate to whomever they match with and are not related to or acquainted with the recipient.

    d. ABO incompatible donor.

      (1) Some transplant centers have a special program for incompatible donors.

      (2) Donation is allowed once the recipient goes through special desensitization therapy to allow for nonrejection of the donor kidney.

    e. Donor swap/paired donation.

      (1) Kidney paired donation allows one incompatible donor/recipient pair to donate to another pair in the same situation.

      (2) The donor of the first pair gives to the recipient of the second, and vice versa (Alliance for Paired Donation, 2009).

  D. Patient age at time of transplantation.

    1. Ages < 1:   0%.

    2. Ages 1 to 4:   18.5%.

    3. Ages 5 to 9:   17.5%.

    4. Ages 10 to 14: 28.3%.

    5. Ages 15.to.17: 35.4% (USRDS, 2013, http://www.usrds.org/2013/ref/E_tx_process_13.xls).

  E. Preemptive transplant versus the need for dialysis prior to transplant.

    1. Transplantation may be the first mode of therapy for some patients.

    2. Preemptive transplants occur more frequently in children because of parents' and patients' desire to avoid dialysis when a living donor is available.

    3. Transplantation is actively promoted by pediatric nephrology centers.

    4. Many centers want pediatric transplant recipients to weigh a minimum of 10 kg.

    5. Morbidity is lower for children with transplantation than with dialysis therapy.

  F. United Network for Organ Sharing (UNOS) and Organ Procurement and Transplant Network (OPTN).

    1. UNOS was awarded the OPTN contract in 1986; it was renewed in 2013.

    2. Established membership standards for transplant centers and organ procurement organizations (OPOs).

    3. Established equitable organ allocation system based on a point system consisting of:

      a. ABO match.

      b. HLA matching.

      c. Pediatric status.

      d. Time waiting on list.

      e. Level of preformed antibodies.

      f. Need for other organ transplants at the same time.

      g. Previous organ donor.

      h. Zero mismatch share nationally ONLY if the calculated panel reactive antibody (CPRA) ≥ 20 (Andreoni, 2013).

    4. Monitors distribution of all organs across the U.S.

    5. Maintains scientific registries.

    6. Facilitates organ placement throughout the U.S.

  G. Patient/graft survival statistics.

    1. Living donor graft survival rate is 85.7 % at 5 years posttransplantation.

    2. Deceased donor graft survival rate is 78.4% at 5 years posttransplantation (NAPTRCS 2010 Annual Report).

  H. Evaluation for transplantation.

    1. ABO grouping determines compatible blood type(s) for a donor kidney for a particular recipient (see Table 1.9).

2. Histocompatibility testing looks at proteins called human leukocyte antigens (HLAs) found on the surface of nearly every cell in the human body.
   a. HLAs are found in large amounts on the surface of white blood cells.
   b. They tell the immune system the difference between native body tissue and foreign substances.
3. Calculated panel reactive antibodies (CPRA).
   a. The CPRA is blood testing that is performed on the donated kidney to determine the presence of preformed antibodies to the human leukocyte antigens (HLA).
   b. It is used in the allocation of donated kidneys as a measure of sensitization level.
   c. The CPRA estimates the percentage of donors that would be incompatible with the candidate (OPTN, 2012).
4. A crossmatch is done prior to every transplant to be sure the recipient does not have preformed antibodies to the donor (called a positive crossmatch).
5. Basic lab studies include, but are not limited to:
   a. Chemistries.
   b. Hematology.
   c. Coagulation studies.
   d. Urine studies.
   e. ABO compatibility.
   f. Monthly antibody screening.
   g. Histocompatibility testing.
6. Viral surveillance and screening includes, but is not limited to:
   a. Human Immunodeficiency Virus (HIV).
   b. Hepatitis B and C.
   c. Epstein-Barr virus (EBV).
   d. Cytomegalovirus (CMV).
   e. Varicella zoster virus (VZV).
   f. Measles, mumps, and rubella titers (MMR) at most centers.
7. Evaluations for infections. The following infections are tested for or assessed for prior to transplantation. Variations exist among centers regarding whether or not to transplant patients with HIV, Hepatitis B, or Hepatitis C. All infections are treated and cleared prior to the initiation of immunosuppressive therapy.
   a. Tuberculosis.
   b. HIV.
   c. Hepatitis B and C.
   d. Dental infections.
   e. Urinary tract infections.
   f. Sinuses.
   g. Skin.
8. Immunizations must be up to date prior to transplantation to assist in infection prevention posttransplantation.

Table 1.9

Compatible Blood Types for a Donor Kidney

Recipient	Donor
A	A, O
B	B, O
O	O
AB	A, B, O, AB

   a. All immunizations should be up to date for age prior to transplantation.
   b. Live virus vaccines should be administered at least 1 to 2 months prior to transplantation (Avery & Michaels, 2008).
9. Evaluation of the urinary system. Urological issues must be evaluated and necessary repairs of urinary tract abnormalities must be made. These could include:
   a. Ureterovesical or ureteropelvic junction obstruction.
   b. Vesicoureteral reflux.
   c. Intermittent catheterization for neurogenic bladder.
   d. Bladder augmentation.
   e. Creation of a Mitrofanoff channel that is used for catheterization.
   f. Removal of duplicated systems.
10. Nephrectomies may be indicated prior to transplantation in certain conditions.
   a. Polycystic kidney disease.
   b. Uncontrolled hypertension.
   c. Congenital nephrotic syndrome.
   d. Denys-Drash syndrome – a disorder with three main parts: kidney disease present at birth, Wilm's tumor, and malformation of the sexual organs.
   e. Severe reflux.
   f. High output kidney diseases.
   g. Severe uncontrollable proteinuria.
11. Evaluation of the cardiovascular system. *Note*: Transplantation may be delayed or cancelled without adequate cardiac function.
   a. Determination of adequate cardiac function.
   b. Assurance that the iliac vasculature is patent.
   c. Assessment for the absence of vascular disease.
   d. Evaluation for hypertension and left ventricular hypertrophy (LVH).
      (1) Determine the cause of HTN and treat appropriately.

(2) Hypertension posttransplantation can cause irreversible damage to the graft.

12. Evaluation of the respiratory system. *Note:* Severe pulmonary disease may preclude a patient from receiving a kidney transplant. Patients are evaluated for:
    a. Asthma.
    b. Bronchopulmonary dysplasia (BPD).
    c. Tuberculosis (TB).
    d. Smoking – teens need to be encouraged to stop smoking.

13. Evaluation of the endocrine system may include assessing for:
    a. Diabetes.
    b. Hyperparathyroidism.

14. Evaluation of the digestive system may assess for:
    a. Active ulcer disease.
    b. Esophageal disease.
    c. Liver disease.
    d. Portal hypertension.
    e. Gastroparesis.

15. Adequate nutrition prior to transplantation is vital in order to:
    a. Prevent metabolic disturbances.
    b. Prevent growth retardation.
    c. Prevent malnutrition.
    d. Promote healing.

16. Children should be assessed for growth and development. Evaluate for and correct the following prior to transplant.
    a. Poor or inadequate nutrition.
    b. Inadequate dialysis.
    c. Anemia.
    d. Anorexia.
    e. Chronic acidosis.
    f. Maximize growth potential pretransplantation with the use of growth hormone therapy.

17. Neuropsychological evaluation is needed prior to transplantation.
    a. The recipient's age determines the process for evaluation.
    b. The evaluation should include assessment for anything that could preclude successful long-term graft survival.
    c. This may include, but is not limited to:
       (1) Mental function.
       (2) Neurologic abnormalities.
       (3) Psychomotor delay.
       (4) Seizures.
       (5) Psychiatric disorders.
       (6) Emotional disorders.
       (7) Nonadherence.

18. Malignancies.
    a. A child must be malignancy free for 1 to 2 years prior to transplantation.
    b. This may vary from center to center; the required length may vary depending on the type of malignancy.

19. A complete dental exam should be performed prior to transplantation.
    a. The teeth and gums should be evaluated prior to transplantation.
    b. Needed dental work must be completed prior to transplant.
    c. The presence of infection may lead to life threatening illness posttransplantation.
    d. Written documentation from the dentist regarding the child's dental status should be obtained.

I. Patient and family education.
   1. Education of patient and caregiver is based on the patient's age and developmental stage.
   2. Education of parent and caregiver should be done at the 5th to 6th grade reading level.
   3. The parent and caregiver may need to be assessed for ability to read or other cognitive dysfunction.
   4. Topics to include.
      a. Pretransplant care.
      b. Intraoperative care and risks.
      c. Postoperative care and risks.

J. The transplant surgery.
   1. The location of allograft is based on patient's size.
      a. Smaller children may have the kidney placed intraperitoneally.
      b. Most kidneys will be placed extraperitoneally in the lower right anterior iliac fossa.
   2. The length of surgery varies based on patient's size and condition, but typically lasts around 4 hours.
   3. Most transplant centers use some type of immunosuppressive therapy starting the day of surgery.
      a. This practice varies from center to center and may even start prior to surgery.
      b. Decisions are based on the patient's cause of kidney failure or if it is an ABO incompatible transplant.
   4. The blood pressure and volume status of every child is closely monitored.
      a. Most children go to the intensive care unit for at least 1 night posttransplantation to closely monitor their fluid and electrolyte status and balance.
      b. Blood pressure is closely monitored to maintain central venous pressure (CVP) between 15 and 20 mmHg at the time of kidney reperfusion.
      c. This is to maintain intravascular integrity and to keep the allograft well perfused.
      d. Allograft thrombosis is one of the leading causes of graft failure early on posttransplantation (Ponticelli et al., 2009).

K. Perioperative/immediate posttransplant care of the pediatric kidney transplant recipient includes, but is not limited to:
   1. Maintenance of cardiac function and adequate circulation.
   2. Maintenance of pulmonary function and adequate respirations.
   3. Maintenance of fluid and electrolyte balance.
   4. Prevention of infection.
   5. Monitoring immunosuppressive therapy.
   6. Monitoring for constipation or diarrhea.
   7. Monitoring for pain.
   8. Monitoring for signs and symptoms of rejection.
   9. Education of patient and family (Counts, 2008; Cupples & Ohler, 2008).

L. Posttransplant and discharge planning care.
   1. All patients and their families and primary caregivers require education.
   2. This education should include, but is not limited to:
      a. Medications: uses, side effects, dosing, storage, etc.
      b. Signs and symptoms of rejection.
      c. Signs and symptoms of infection.
      d. Routine follow-up care with the transplant center and the primary care physician.
      e. Activity level in the first 4 to 6 weeks postoperatively and long term.
         (1) Most centers limit contact sports for kidney transplant recipients, but this varies.
         (2) Some centers recommend some type of protective covering or garment over the allograft area to protect it during contact sports.
      f. Who to call and when to call.
         (1) Contact numbers of appropriate members of the transplant team to reach for needs, concerns, illness, etc.
         (2) Also need a list of "what to call for" and things to watch for.
      g. Home needs and arrangements.
         (1) Will the child need some type of home health care or IV therapy?
         (2) Will the child need dialysis for a short period of time in the case of delayed graft function?
      h. Diet and fluid needs.
         (1) Specific dietary restrictions and oral fluid intake. A gastrostomy tube (G-tube) or a nasogastric tube (NG tube) may be required for sufficient intake.
         (2) Dehydration can lead to elevated creatinine or allograft thrombosis in the early posttransplant period.
      i. Basic childhood wellness care.
         (1) Maintain routine well-child care, including vaccinations and dental care prior to transplantation.

(2) The length of time until a child can resume routine dental care or immunizations varies, but it is usually around 3 to 6 months following the transplantation. *Note*: Live vaccines are not indicated in immunosuppressed individuals.

M. Posttransplant complications can be divided into early/short-term and late/long-term.
   1. Early or short-term complications.
      a. Delayed graft function can be caused by prolonged storage time, prolonged warm ischemia time, acute tubular necrosis (ATN), or severe rejection.
      b. Hyperacute rejection happens minutes to hours posttransplantation.
      c. Acute rejection happens days to weeks posttransplant.
      d. Thrombosis of the renal artery or renal vein. Small children are at the highest risk for thrombosis due to low blood flow rates compared to the blood flow rates of the donor.
      e. Obstruction.
      f. Bleeding at the surgical anastamosis sites.
      g. Infections of any type.
      h. Urine leak may be caused by a ureteral leak or disruption, or from the bladder.
      i. Incisional/wound problems like dehiscence, perinephric hematomas, urinomas, lymphoceles, or abscess.
      j. Graft rupture.
   2. Late or long-term complications.
      a. Hyperlipidemia can be caused by medications, diet, or genetics.
      b. Infections are screened for frequently in pediatric patients.
         (1) Bacterial infections can include pneumonia, or urinary tract.
         (2) Viral infections account for 25% to 30% of the infections in children posttransplant.
      c. Children are five times more likely to develop primary viral infections due to lack of exposure pretransplantation, and thus lack of immunity. Viral infections can include:
         (1) Epstein-Barr virus (EBV): a seronegative status pretransplant is associated with a higher risk of posttransplant lymphoproliferative disease (PTLD).
         (2) Cytomegalovirus (CMV).
         (3) Varicella zoster virus (VZV) can be severe and have many complications including encephalitis, pneumonitis, hepatic dysfunction, and even death.
      d. Wound infections.
      e. Opportunistic infections such as *Pneumocystis carinii* pneumonia (PCP).

N. Disease recurrence.
    1. Some primary diseases have a high recurrence rate posttransplantation and must be monitored carefully.
    2. These could include:
        a. Membranoproliferative glomerulonephritis involving the basement membrane and the mesangium.
        b. Membranous glomerulonephritis involves the basement membrane but not the mesangium.
        c. Lupus.
        d. IgA nephropathy.
        e. Atypical HUS.
        f. FSGS.
        g. Primary hyperoxaluria – the best therapy is combined liver and kidney transplant

O. Malignancies.
    1. May occur posttransplantation.
    2. Many medications used to prevent rejection increase risk of cancers/malignancies posttransplant, including:
        a. Posttransplant lymphoproliferative disease (PTLD).
        b. Lymphoma.
        c. Skin cancers.

P. Hypertension.
    1. Requires monitoring and treatment to prevent damage to the allograft.
    2. May occur early or late posttransplantation.

Q. Cardiac disease.
    1. In recent years, cardiac disease is more common in children.
    2. Requires awareness and monitoring.

R. Nutrition.
    1. The patient's nutritional status requires monitoring.
    2. Intensive education is essential.
    3. Posttransplant interventions are required in children.
        a. Hypophosphatemia or hypercalcemia due to secondary hyperparathyroidism may require supplements.
        b. Hypokalemia from pretransplant diet restrictions coupled with normal urinary output posttransplantation may respond to liberalizing the diet.
        c. Dehydration from years of fluid restriction while on kidney replacement therapy (KRT) is common.
        d. Increased appetite due to improved kidney function and the use of steroids may lead to sudden, excessive weight gains.

S. Diabetes posttransplantation may be due to steroids and calcineurin inhibitor use.

T. Growth and development posttransplantation.
    1. The use of steroids and the patient's age at time of transplantation impact posttransplant growth. Children under the age of 6 demonstrate the best outcomes regarding growth.
    2. Factors affecting growth and development posttransplantation.
        a. Poor allograft function can inhibit growth.
        b. Growth can be improved by the use of growth hormone (GH). Beginning GH is usually delayed for 1 to 2 years after the transplant.

U. Dental care is imperative posttransplantation.
    1. Healthy teeth and gums is the goal.
    2. The use of antibiotic prophylaxis is center specific.

V. Nonadherence with the medical therapy posttransplantation is quite problematic, especially with the adolescent.
    1. Factors influencing adherence.
        a. Misunderstanding of dose changes.
        b. Belief that medications are not helpful.
        c. Disorganized family structure.
        d. The adolescent's need for control and lack of understanding of long-term consequences.
        e. Complexity of medication regimen.
        f. Body image changes.
    2. Tips to assist with patient and family adherence.
        a. Simplification of medication administration and dosage times.
        b. Ongoing education.
        c. Frequent clinic visits.
        d. Behavior modification.
        e. Counseling.

W. Psychosocial issues after transplant occur for many reasons.
    1. Return to school, which equates to "work" for children.
    2. Body image changes.
    3. Financial issues for parent(s) resulting from having to be away from work and/or home for long periods of time.
    4. Emotional issues for both the patient and parent(s) related to the parents missing work, and/or being gone from home and other children for long periods of time.
    5. The cost of medications as well as extended stays away from home.
    6. Keeping the child insured to cover medical expenses.
    7. Transitioning a pediatric patient to adult care.

X. Rejection of the transplanted kidney.
1. Hyperacute.
    a. Occurs within minutes or up to 24 hours following surgery.
    b. Difficult to treat and is often irreversible.
    c. Less common with the improved cross-matching techniques now used.
2. Accelerated.
    a. Occurs within 3 to 5 days posttransplantation.
    b. Difficult to treat.
3. Acute.
    a. More common in first 6 months after transplantation, but can occur later.
    b. One of leading causes of re-admission following surgery.
4. Chronic allograft nephropathy, also known as chronic rejection, is the most common cause of graft loss in children (Counts, 2008; Cupples & Ohler, 2008).

Y. Medications.
1. Used to prevent rejection, infection, and to protect the stomach from immunosuppressants.
2. Commonly used medications to prevent rejection.
    a. Immunosuppressants to prevent rejection of the allograft.
    b. Calcineurin inhibitors such as tacrolimus (Prograf®) and cyclosporine work by suppressing the activation of T lymphocytes.
    c. Antiproliferative agents/antimetabolites, such as azathioprine and mycophenolic acid, suppress T-cell and B-cell proliferation.
    d. mTOR inbitors, including rapamycin or everolimus, work by inhibiting kinase.
    e. Corticosteroids such as prednisone or methyl-prednisolone are complex and affect multiple areas. They were the first generation of immunosuppressants marketed.
    f. Rejection therapies used at the time of the transplant as induction therapy, or later as therapy to treat severe rejection, include basilixamab, alemtuzumab, and antithymocyte globulin.
3. Antiviral medications are prescribed to prevent the development of viral infections after kidney transplant.
    a. The majority of children are not exposed to Epstein-Barr virus (EBV) or cytomegalovirus (CMV).
    b. Most adults are EBV or CMV positive before their transplants.
    c. Medications such as acyclovir, valacyclovir, ganciclovir, or valganciclovir, are used to prevent these diseases.
4. Antifungal agents help prevent fungal infections after transplant. These may include clotrimazole, nystatin, or fluconazole.
5. Antibiotics help prevent opportunistic infections; may include sulfamethoxazole, cefazolin, and pentamidine (especially in a patient with sulfa allergies).
6. Proton pump inhibitors or H2 blockers are commonly used for side effects of the antimetabolites and large doses of steroids; may include ranitidine, famotidine, omeprazole, or lansoprazole.
7. Antihypertensive medications may include beta blockers, ACE inhibitors, or angiotensin II blockers. The different classes are typically used at different time frames posttransplantation (Counts, 2008; Cuddles, 2008).

II. Peritoneal dialysis (PD) in pediatric patients.

(For more information, see Peritoneal Dialysis chapter: Module 3, Chapter 4).

A. Indications for PD.
1. PD is the treatment of choice for patients who are ages 0 to 4 years (75% vs. 25%) (USRDS, 2013; Warady, et al, 2012).
2. PD is common in children < 13 years of age; the 2012 Annual Data Report of USRDS showed hemodialysis is the most common modality of children 0 to 19 years of age (Mak & Warady, 2013).
3. The peritoneal membrane in children is very large in relation to their body surface area.

B. Types of PD.
1. Continuous ambulatory peritoneal dialysis (CAPD).
    a. Exchanges take place during the day.
    b. There is a higher incidence of peritonitis in children.
    c. Requires a caregiver to perform the treatment unless the child is older or an adolescent.
    d. Exchanges do not require the use of a machine.
    e. Exchanges occur 4 to 6 times per day and are performed by patient and/or caregiver. These exchanges typically require that the caregiver and/or parent of patient perform.
    f. Often used in pediatrics as a backup treatment in case of a power outage and/or emergency.
    g. Requires the child to tolerate longer dwell times, depending on peritoneal membrane characteristics (determined by Peritoneal Equilibration Test).
2. Continuous cycling peritoneal dialysis (CCPD).
    a. Treatments are done using a machine programmed with the prescription and cycles desired.
    b. Settings are programmed for inflow volume and time, dwell time, outflow time, and number of cycles.

c. The automated system allows the child to receive treatments for 8 to 12 hours each night.

d. The cycler accounts for each cycle ultrafiltration (UF) and total UF of treatment.

e. The cycler is used in hospital and home settings for dialysis.

f. Typical treatment duration is 8 to 12 hours nightly.

g Cyclers allow for a daytime exchange if ordered by the nephrologist, APRN, or PA.

h. Some cyclers have electronic data recording capabilities (data card, modem).

3. Manual peritoneal dialysis (Alparslan et al., 2012).

a. Used in neonates or small infants when volume of fill is less than 50 to 100 mL/cycle.

b. 20 to 40 mL/kg of dialysate is warmed to 37°C, infused over 10 to 15 minutes, allowed to dwell 10 to 20 minutes, and drained over 10 to 15 minutes in continuous cycles.

c. Closed system volume sets (such as Dialy-Nate®, http://www.utahmed.com) allow for manual dialysis procedures.

d. Time-intensive procedure requiring every 30 minutes to every hour interventions by the bedside nurse, which frequently is done in the intensive care unit (ICU) setting.

e. Requires special training and competencies in care of the neonate or infant on peritoneal dialysis for hospital staff performing procedures.

f. Tubing change per manufacturer's recommendations.

C. Peritoneal treatment.

1. Initiation of peritoneal dialysis in pediatric patient (Warady et al., 2012).

2. Initial fill volumes are approximately 10 mL/kg (Warady et al., 2004).

3. Goal fill volumes for children are 1100 mL/m² (Warady et al., 2004).

4. Manual dialysis exchanges are done for patients who have a fill volume less than 50 to 100 mL.

5. Continuous cycling peritoneal dialysis (CCPD) using a cycler can be initiated when the fill volume is greater than 50 to 100 mL, or per cycler manufacturer recommendations.

D. Access placement.

1. PD catheter placement should preferably occur at least 2 weeks prior to initiation of dialysis to allow for adequate healing of the catheter tunnel and exit site.

2. The placement of a chronic PD catheter occurs in the operating room (OR), allowing for an omentectomy and visualization of the peritoneal space.

3. Preoperative bowel preparation should occur to decrease risk of bacterial translocation and catheter malposition after placement.

4. Administration of an antibiotic prior to incision time has been shown to decrease early infectious complications following PD catheter placement. Center-specific susceptibility patterns should be considered when choosing the antibiotic (Warady et al., 2012).

5. Catheter placement should be performed by a surgeon or nephrologist skilled in PD catheter placement.

6. Catheter placement can be performed using the open surgical technique or the laparoscopic technique.

7. The external cuff should be placed 2 cm from the exit site to prevent cuff extrusion.

8. The location of exit site should take into consideration the patient's belt line, diaper line, and presence of stomas (e.g., gastrostomy, vesicostomy, colostomy, ureterostomy).

9. A double cuff Tenckhoff® catheter with an exit-site orientation lateral or downward is preferred.

10. There should be no sutures at exit site as they increase the risk of bacterial colonization.

11. Fibroblast ingrowth of Dacron® cuff is sufficient to anchor the catheter.

12. The catheter should be anchored close to the exit site to prevent trauma to the tunnel. Tape, dressing, PD belts, or commercial anchoring devices may be used.

13. Utilization of surgical glue.

a. Fibrin glue can be applied to the peritoneal cuff suture to prevent early dialysate leakage in patients where the catheter will be used for dialysis shortly after placement (Warady et al., 2012, p. S36).

b. Dermabond® can be used at the exit site when leaks occur and/or when the catheter will be used for dialysis shortly after placement.

E. Exit-site care.

1. Early exit-site care.

a. A sterile dressing should be applied until the catheter is well healed.

(1) This typically takes a minimum of 2 weeks but can take up to 6 weeks.

(2) A healed exit site is "when the skin around the exit site looks normal without gaping."

b. The sterile dressing should be changed weekly by trained health care personnel to avoid manipulation of catheter and trauma to exit site and tunnel during healing phase. The dressing should only be changed more frequently if the exit site is soiled, damp, and/or dressing is not intact.

c. The site should be cleansed in a sterile fashion using a nonirritating, nontoxic agent; do not use povidone iodine or hydrogen peroxide as they can be damaging to the granulation tissue in the sinus tract (Warady et al., 2012).

   d. The dressing can consist of sterile gauze and antibiotic cream or chlorhexidine gluconate (CHG) impregnated patches with a sterile, transparent dressing.

   e. The catheter should be allowed to fall into a natural position and be reinforced with an anchor just below the exit site to prevent trauma to the tunnel.

2. Chronic exit-site care.

   a. The exit site should be cleansed daily with sterile gauze and a nonirritating, nontoxic antiseptic agent. Gentamicin cream, mupirocin cream, or medihoney are recommended as acceptable agents (Warady et al., 2012, p. S40, S41).

   b. The exit site should be assessed daily by the caregiver and/or patient for redness, drainage, swelling, scabbing, or other infectious signs.

   c. Topical antibiotic cream should be applied daily to exit site.

   d. The catheter should be anchored just below the exit site using tape, dressing, PD belt, or other commercial anchoring device.

F. Complications of peritoneal dialysis in infants and children.

1. Infection is a major complication of PD: urinary tract infections or peritonitis.

   a. Infection is the most frequent cause of hospitalization in children (USRDS, 2013).

   b. It is the leading cause of modality change in pediatric patients (NAPRTCS, 2011).

   c. For a comprehensive set of recommendations, refer to "Consensus Guidelines for the Prevention and Treatment of Catheter-Related Infections and Peritonitis in Pediatric Patients Receiving Peritoneal Dialysis: 2012 Update." http://www.pdiconnect.com/content/32/Supplement_2/S32.full.pdf+html

2. Mechanical complications.

   a. Inflow obstruction can be caused by fibrin or blood clots in the PD catheter.

     (1) This can be treated with a normal saline flush and/or the use of alteplase in the catheter to break down the clot in the line.

     (2) It can also be caused by a kink in the catheter or a clamp engaged on the line.

   b. Outflow obstruction is most commonly caused by constipation, catheter kinking, catheter malposition, or obstruction by fibrin, blood clots, or omentum.

     (1) An appropriate bowel regimen can correct constipation.

     (2) Fibrin or blood clots can be treated with a normal saline flush and/or use of alteplase in catheter to break down clot in line.

     (3) Catheter malposition and omentum entrapment require surgical intervention to correct.

   c. Hernias are a common complication in infants and neonates on PD.

     (1) The most common sites of hernia formation are the inguinal canals with or without patent processus vaginalis, the umbilicus, the linea alba, the exit site, and other sites of prior surgical incision (Warady et al., 2012).

     (2) The majority of hernias require surgical repair.

     (3) Postoperatively, these patients should be maintained on low volume PD with empty or reduced dwell during the daytime (Warady et al., 2012).

   d. Hydrothorax is an uncommon complication of PD and can be diagnosed on chest x-ray.

     (1) Shows a right-sided pleural effusion.

     (2) PD must be stopped until leakage has resolved.

3. Prescription-related complications.

   a. Inadequate solute clearance can occur when fill volumes are either too large or too small, dialysis time is insufficient, or dwell times are not applicable to patient's peritoneal membrane characteristics, determined by PET test.

   b. Hypervolemia.

     (1) Can occur when the fill volumes are insufficient, dextrose is insufficient, or dialysis time is insufficient.

     (2) This can result in hypertension, respiratory distress, and edema.

   c. Hypovolemia.

     (1) Can occur when:

       (a) The dextrose ordered is producing excessive ultrafiltration (UF).

       (b) The patient has increased fluid losses secondary to vomiting, diarrhea, large urine output, or increased insensible losses.

       (c) The patient is not taking in enough fluid throughout the day.

     (2) This can result in hypotension, weakness, fainting, or other complications related to hypotension.

4. Other complications (Warady et al., 2012).

   a. Peritoneal membrane failure.

     (1) Adequate solute removal and ultrafiltration are not achieved.

     (2) A change in PD prescription and/or solutions is often warranted.

     (3) Change in modality may occur as a result of membrane failure.

b. Encapsulating peritoneal sclerosis (Honda et al., 2010).

  (1) An uncommon but the most serious complication of PD resulting in a 30% mortality rate.

  (2) Caused by a thickening of the peritoneal membrane and vessels, resulting in calcification of the mesothelial layer.

  (3) Signs and symptoms include abdominal pain, nausea, vomiting, fatigue, loss of appetite, constipation, diarrhea, abdominal mass, ascites, weight loss, low-grade fever, and resistance to erythropoiesis-stimulating agents (ESAs).

  (4) Risk factors include:

    (a) The amount of time treated with PD with the incidence increasing to 20% after 8 years of therapy.

    (b) Recurrent bacterial peritonitis or hypertonic glucose exposure.

  (5) Treatment includes discontinuation of PD, bowel rest, and immunosuppressive therapy.

c. Hemoperitoneum.

  (1) This is the presence of blood in the PD effluent, which is a benign complication.

  (2) Small amounts of blood in the effluent bag can color the effluent from blood tinged to bright red.

5. Other barriers to PD (Chavers et al., 2007).

  a. Malnutrition.

  b. Vitamin D deficiency.

G. Peritoneal dialysis training content (Warady et al., 2011).

1. Theory.

  a. Functions of the kidney.

  b. Overview of PD (osmosis and diffusion).

  c. Fluid balance (include the relationship between weight and blood pressure).

  d. Use of different strengths and types of dialysis fluids.

  e. Prevention of infection.

2. Practical.

  a. Handwashing.

  b. Aseptic technique.

  c. Dialysis therapy – machine or manual exchanges (step-by-step procedure guide).

  d. Emergency measures for contamination.

  e. Troubleshooting or problem-solving alarms on the cycler.

  f. Blood pressure monitoring and recording.

  g. Weight monitoring and recording.

  h. Exit-site care.

3. Complications.

  a. Signs, symptoms, and treatment of peritonitis.

  b. Signs, symptoms, and treatment of exit site and tunnel infections.

  c. Drain problems (constipation, fibrin).

  d. Fluid balance (hypertension, hypotension).

  e. Other (leaks, pain).

4. Other.

  a. Recordkeeping.

  b. Administration of medications.

  c. Dietary management.

  d. Ordering and managing supplies.

  e. Managing life with PD (e.g., school, sports, holidays).

  f. Contacting the hospital or dialysis center, making clinic visits, and arranging home visits.

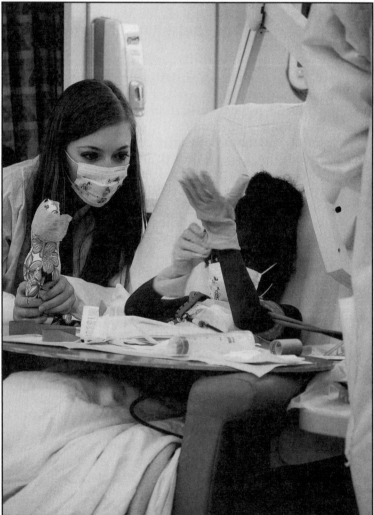

Play therapy can facilitate trust, especially for younger children.

Photo courtesy of Robin Davis.

III. Hemodialysis in children.

A. The majority of children with CKD stage 5 receive dialytic therapy prior to transplantation.
   1. 50% receive maintenance HD as a bridge to transplantation.
   2. Pediatric centers were created to meet unique demands of pediatric patients with CKD stage 5.
   3. Developmental, nutritional, and social needs must be considered when treating children.
   4. Considerable resources are required but have shown increased survival and rehabilitation of children with CKD stage 5 (Muller & Goldstein, 2011).

B. Vascular access.
   (For more information, see Module 3, Chapter 4, Vascular Access.)
   1. Guidance for hemodialysis in pediatric patients with CKD stage 5.
      a. In 1987, the North American Pediatric Renal Transplant Cooperative Study (NAPRTCS) was organized to collect data on all pediatric transplants in the United States.
         (1) In 1992, the study expanded to include pediatric patients on dialysis.
         (2) In 1994, included patients with CKD with glomerular filtration rates (GFR) < 30 mL/min/1.73 m^2 (NAPRTCS, 2011).
      b. In 1997, the National Kidney Foundation (NKF) established the Dialysis Outcomes Quality Initiative (DOQI) Clinical Practice Guidelines, but with no pediatric guidance for vascular access.
         (1) In 2006, the guidelines were updated to the NKF Kidney Disease Outcomes Quality Initiative (KDOQI).
         (2) A section was created for clinical practice recommendations for vascular access in pediatric patients (NKF, 2006B).
      c. In 1999, the American Society of Pediatric Nephrologists (ASPN) published a paper on the optimal care of the pediatric ESRD patient (Andreoli et al., 2005).
      d. In 2003, the Centers for Medicare and Medicaid Services (CMS) created the National Vascular Access Improvement Initiative (NVAII), later to become the Fistula First Breakthrough Initiative (FFBI) in 2005.
      e. The International Pediatric Fistula First Initiative (IPFFI) began as collaboration with ESRD Networks 9 and 10 and the Midwest Pediatric Nephrology Consortium in 2005 (Chand & Valentini, 2008).
      f. Patients with an estimated GFR < 30 mL/min/1.73 m^2 (CKD stage 4), or expected to reach CKD stage 5 within 6 to 12 months, should be educated on options for kidney replacement therapy: PD, home HD, in-center HD, transplantation, and palliative care (Manook & Calder, 2012).
      g. Early referral for placement of a permanent dialysis access is essential (Manook & Calder, 2012).
   2. Vascular access options.
      a. An AVF is preferred for children who weigh less than 20 kg or if transplant is more than 1 year away (Mak & Warady, 2013; NKF, 2006b). Advantages of an AVF include:
         (1) Higher access survival rates (Ma et al., 2013).
         (2) Lower infection rates.
         (3) Significant decrease in hospitalizations.
      b. The AVG should be avoided if possible (Manook & Calder, 2012).
         (1) Preadolescent low blood pressure causes clotting.
         (2) Used only if an AVF is not possible.
      c. Avoid central venous catheters (CVC), if possible, because of:
         (1) Higher infection rates.
         (2) Higher hospitalization rates.
         (3) Stenosis (Chand & Valentini, 2008).
         (4) Thrombosis (Chand & Valentini, 2008).
         (5) Lower albumin rates (Fadrowski et al., 2006).
         (6) Lower hemoglobin rates (Fadrowski et al., 2006).
      d. A CVC could be appropriate when (NKF, 2006b):
         (1) There is a lack of surgical expertise; refer to a surgeon who performs adult access placement.
         (2) The patient's size is too small for an AVF/AVG.
         (3) Bridge to early transplantation (< 1 year).
         (4) Bridge to peritoneal dialysis (PD).
         (5) Bridge to hemodialysis when a PD catheter has to be removed due to peritonitis.
   3. Vein preservation (Manook & Calder, 2012).
      a. Nondominant arm first for dialysis access. Start distally, work proximally.
      b. Upper limbs before lower limbs.
      c. Blood draws/IVs in dorsal veins of hands.
      d. Prevent the use of a peripherally inserted central catheter (PICC) line in any patient with CKD stage 2 or greater to preserve access for later dialysis.
   4. Identified barriers to access types.
      a. AV fistula (Chand & Valentini, 2008).
         (1) Inadequate referral times.
         (2) Poor communication between the nephrologist and surgeon.
         (3) Patient and/or family resistance.
         (4) Arterial/venous spasm.
         (5) Primary AV fistula failure.

(6) Hypercoagulable state.

(7) Long time to maturation: 4 to 6 months.

(8) No pediatric surgeon.

(9) Size of the patient's vasculature.

b. AV graft (Chand & Valentini, 2008).

(1) Clotting.

(2) Infection.

(3) Limited life use.

c. Central venous catheters (Chand & Valentini, 2008).

(1) Central vein stenosis.

(2) High infection rates.

(3) Clotting.

5. Monitoring (Chand et al., 2009).

a. Physical exam weekly.

b. Difficulty with needle insertion.

c. Decrease in blood flow – more negative arterial prepump pressures.

6. Surveillance (Chand et al., 2009).

a. Ultrasound dilution technique or Doppler ultrasound monthly.

b. Access recirculation studies monthly.

7. Referral for intervention.

a. Access recirculation > 20%.

b. Ultrasound dilution – access flow < 650 mL/min; abnormal Doppler ultrasound.

c. Formation of aneurysm or pseudoaneurysm.

C. Fluid removal in children is extremely important to prevent long-term consequences.

1. Volume overload contributes to:

a. Expanded extracellular volume (ECV).

b. Cardiovascular risk, such as hypertension, left ventricular hypertrophy (LVH), and arrhythmias.

c. Hypoalbuminemia.

d. Anemia; i.e., hypervolemia dilutes the hemoglobin (Hgb) and hematocrit (Hct).

e. Inflammation.

f. Bowel wall edema, increased gut permeability, and increased plasma endotoxin levels (Reyes-Bahamonde et al., 2013).

g. Dyspnea, coughing, and/or increased respiratory rate.

h. Hypoxia due to pulmonary vascular congestion.

i. Rales and wheezing.

j. Physical inactivity.

2. Volume is a nondose related component of adequacy.

a. Accurate assessment of the patient's intravascular volume during the HD treatment should be provided to optimize ultrafiltration (KDOQI Table 15.4 8.4, NKF 2006 updates).

b. It is a CMS Condition for Coverage to manage the patient's volume status under the "Patient plan of care" condition (§ 494.90(a)(1) http://www.cms.gov/Regulations-and-Guidance/Legislation/CFCsAndCoPs

c. For pediatric patients weighing less than 35 kg, blood volume monitoring during hemodialysis should be available in order to evaluate body weight changes for gains in muscle weight vs. fluid overload (CMS V504) (see Table 1.10).

d. In evaluating volume status, blood pressure (BP) should be the lower of 90% of normal for age/weight/height or 130/80.

3. Equipment needed for hematocrit-based blood volume monitoring.

a. A Clinical Laboratory Improvement Amendments (CLIA)-exempt noninvasive portable monitoring device (e.g., Crit Line™).

(1) Plugged into electrical power.

(2) A disposable one-time use sterile blood chamber attached between the arterial end of the dialyzer and the arterial tubing prior to the initiation of treatment.

b. Integrated device implemented by manufacturer into dialysis machine (e.g., Nikkiso DBB-07 with blood volume monitor with Haemo-Master™).

c. Data retrieval system that includes a printer or wireless transmission to a printer or computer.

4. Description.

a. The monitor neither predicts nor prevents hypotension.

b. Red blood cells (RBCs) have light-absorbing and light-scattering properties. Different light wavelengths transilluminate the blood in the blood chamber, and a lab-equivalent hematocrit is continuously measured photo-optically.

c. The hematocrit is a surrogate for blood volume (Boyle & Sobotka, 2006).

d. [(Start Hct/Current Hct) –1] X 100 = BVΔ%.

e. The monitor does not provide absolute values of blood volume.

f. It provides a continuous measurement of the percent change of blood volume from the initiation of treatment.

g. The hematocrit and the blood volume are inversely related.

h. An increase in the hematocrit from baseline reflects a corresponding decrease in blood volume.

i. If the UF rate exceeds the refilling rate, blood volume contraction occurs, and blood volume percent decreases.

j. If the UF rate is equal to the refilling rate, blood volume percent remains unchanged, even though fluid is being removed.

k. An unchanging blood volume percent indicates that fluid being removed from the vascular compartment is being replenished by fluid from the intracellular and extracellular fluid compartments.

Table 1.10

Evaluating Volume Status

V Tag	Patient Assessment § 494.80	V Tag	Plan of Care § 494.90
V504	BP/fluid management needs	V543	Management of volume status
	Interdialytic BP & weight gain Target Symptoms Value - Euvolemic & BP 130/80		Management of volume status Euvolemic and BP 130/80
V507	Anemia	V547	Achieve and sustain Hgb/Hct
	Volume Bleeding Infection ESA hypo-response		Hgb on ESAs 10-12 g/dL Hgb off ESAs >10 g/dL

Adapted from: Centers for Medicare & Medicaid Services – Version 1.3.

l. A decrease in the hematocrit from baseline, or in the absence of ultrafiltration, reflects a corresponding increase in blood volume.
m. Albumin and normal saline flushes or boluses will dilute the hematocrit, and blood volume percent will increase.
n. It is also possible that albumin will not only increase blood volume due to actual volume infused, but also due to its oncotic influence recruiting fluid from the extracellular compartment to the vascular compartment (Diroll & Hlebovy, 2003).
o. It is possible for fluid to shift from the extracellular compartment more rapidly than the UF rate is removing fluid from the vascular compartment. In this instance, blood volume percent will increase from blood volume at baseline.
p. The monitor also measures continuous real-time lab-equivalent oxygen saturation (Boyle & Sobotka, 2006).

5. Interpretation of oxygen saturation.
   a If the patient has a graft or a fistula, the saturation is read from arterial blood (SaO_2).
   b. A normal SaO_2 is 97%. It is clinically significant if it falls below 90%.
   c. SaO_2 reveals information about pulmonary status.
   d. If patient has a central venous catheter (CVC), the saturation is read from venous blood (SvO_2 or $ScvO_2$).
   e. A normal SvO_2 is 75% with a range from 60% to 80%.
   f. SvO_2 reveals information about cardiac status.
   g. Supplemental oxygen may be prescribed by cannula or mask for SaO_2 of less than 90%, or for SvO_2 of less than 60%.

6. Factors affecting SaO_2. The SaO_2 reflects the body's supply side. Certain conditions impair this supply system, including:
   a. Decreased cardiac output, such as in heart failure and shock.
   b. Inadequate binding of oxygen to hemoglobin (e.g., nitrate or nitrate therapy, sulfonamide therapy, certain anesthetics).
   c. Anemia resulting from inadequate amounts of hemoglobin.
   d. Increased tissue oxygen requirements (e.g., thyroid storm, hyperthermia, prolonged exercise, status epilepticus).
   e. Inability of cells to absorb or use the oxygen they receive (e.g., sepsis).
   f. Hypoventilation, pulmonary vascular congestion, pneumonia; insufficient oxygen crosses the alveolar-capillary membrane.

7. Factors affecting SvO_2. The SvO_2 reflects the body's demand side. There is a balance between available oxygen (supply) and tissue consumption (demand). In patients with a CVC, a 5% to 7% point decrease in SvO_2 has been associated with a decreased BP (Cordtz et al., 2008).
   a. Conditions that raise SvO_2, reflecting lower demand include:
      (1) Anesthesia.
      (2) Chemical paralysis.
      (3) Elevated SaO_2 levels.
      (4) Hypothermia.
      (5) Increased cardiac output.
      (6) Increased hemoglobin level.
      (7) Sedation.

Caveat: If levels are "high" (> 80%) and incongruent with the patient's condition, evaluate the system for air (a malfunctioning air detector may not alarm). A microscopic hole or tear in the CVC is a remote possibility.

    b. Conditions that lower the SvO$_2$, reflecting increased demand for oxygen, include:
- (1) Decreased cardiac output (e.g., possibly related to hypovolemia).
- (2) Cardiogenic shock.
- (3) Decreased hemoglobin level.
- (4) Fever or hyperthermia.
- (5) Reduced SaO$_2$ levels.
- (6) Seizures.
- (7) Septic shock.
- (8) Shivering.

Caveat: If a child is moving, talking animatedly, or engrossed in an exciting video game, oxygen uptake will be increased and SvO$_2$ will decrease. This is a normal response to activity, and not a cause for alarm. To accurately evaluate decreasing SvO$_2$ levels, the patient should be quiet and calm (Bauer, Reinhart, & Bauer, 2008; Cordtz et al., 2008; West, 2011).

8. Fluid removal during hemodialysis.
   a. The usual goal for fluid removal is ≤ 5% of the child's predialysis weight.
   b. Accurate assessment of the patient's intravascular volume using blood volume monitoring optimizes ultrafiltration in children.
   c. Maximum total blood volume reduction should not exceed 16% change.
   d. The UF rate should be titrated to achieve a targeted blood volume not exceeding an 8% to 12% reduction in measured blood volume in the first hour.
   e. Subsequent hours should result in no more than a 4% to 5% blood volume reduction per hour.
   f. Signs and symptoms of intradialytic hypotension include decreasing SvO$_2$, yawning, headache, hypotension, tachycardia, nausea, vomiting, and restlessness. These symptoms should be treated promptly by decreasing the UF rate for at least 5 minutes. Observe for vascular refilling.
      - (1) If refilling does not occur within 5 to 10 minutes, adjust the desired target loss to reflect a new fluid removal goal.
      - (2) The estimated dry weight (EDW) needs to be adjusted frequently since children should be growing and gaining weight. Conversely, an ill child with an intercurrent infection and decreased appetite could be losing weight.

9. Refill procedure (see Table 1.11) (Rodriguez, 2005).
   a. Note the hematocrit.
   b. Decrease or turn off the UF.
   c. Wait 10 minutes.
   d. Note hematocrit again.
   e. Interpretation.
      - (1) If the hematocrit decreases by 0.5 percentage points or more (example: from 37.5% to 37.0%), then the child has refill. With the UF off, fluid is still able to shift from the extracellular compartment to the intravascular compartment, indicating that the patient is not at the dry weight.
      - (2) If the hematocrit remains unchanged, increases or decreases by 0.4 percentage points or less (example: 37.5% to 37.3%), then there is no refill, indicating that the child is vascularly dry. This can also happen in cases of hypoalbuminemia and/or sepsis – edema is present, but the ability of the extracellular fluid to mobilize is compromised by the disease state.

10. Blood volume monitoring is determined by specific unit policies. See example below (Patel et al., 2007).
    a. Remove 50% of the UF goal in the first hour of treatment, with a maximum blood volume change limited to 8% to 12% in the first hour.
    b. Remove the second 50% of the UF goal in the remaining treatment time, with the maximum change in blood volume limited to 5% per hour in the second, third, and fourth hours.
    c. Assess for plasma refilling weekly, and adjust the dry weight accordingly (Patel et al., 2007).

Table 1.11

Assessment of dry weight based on changes in blood volume, postdialytic vascular compartment refill, and symptoms of hypovolemia

Blood volume reduction	Postdialytic vascular refill	Symptoms of hypovolemia/ postdialysis fatigue	Dry weight change
Yes	No	No	No
Yes	No	Yes	Revise up
Yes	Yes	No	Revise down
Yes	Yes	Yes	Revise down
No	No	No	Revise down

Source: Rodriguez et al., 2005

11. Complications of blood volume monitoring.
    a. Blood leaks.
        (1) Ensure the blood chamber is securely attached to arterial end of dialyzer and tubing.
        (2) Avoid cross-threading.
    b. Inaccurate hematocrit (and hence BVΔ% data) due to air or saline in blood chamber. Ensure it is correctly primed prior to initiation of treatment.
    c. Ignoring rapidly declining BVΔ% or SvO_2 because the child is asymptomatic and the BP is stable.
        (1) A stable BP in the event of BV declination is a result of cardiovascular and neurohormonal compensation.
        (2) If vascular refill is delayed, longer or more frequent treatments may be necessary.
12. Causes of nonvolume related hypotension.
    a. Air embolism.
    b. Infection.
    c. Hypoxia.
    d. Drug reaction (e.g., heparin, iron).
    e. Diminished cardiac reserve (e.g., right heart failure, cardiomyopathy).
    f. Autonomic dysfunction.
    g. Dialysate endotoxin.
    h. Membrane reaction.
    i. Anemia.
    j. Antihypertensives.
    k. Opioid and narcotic analgesics.
    l. Paradoxical effect of some drugs (e.g., albuterol, diphenhydramine).
    m. Hypoglycemia.
    n. Incorrect BP cuff size or placement, cuff over clothing, arm above heart level.
    o. Splanchnic vasodilation due to eating.
    p. Dialysate temperature too high.

D. Pediatric hemodialysis tricks for success.
    1. Estimated blood volume (EBV).
        a. Calculation of the EBV is required and is dependent on the patient's size. The estimated blood volume can be determined by using the following formula:
        EBV = ~ 80 mL/kg
        Example: 80 (mL) x 10 (kg) = 800 mL EBV
        b. Smaller blood tubing is needed. The system should be primed with blood if more than 10% of patient's EBV will be in the circuit.
        c. When the system is primed with blood, discontinue the treatment without returning the blood in the circuit to the patient.
    2. The blood flow rate (BFR).
        a. The BFR can range from 3 to 5 mL/kg/min. This is especially important with infants and small children.
        b. Calculate the maximum BFR using the formula: 2.5 mL x wt (kg) + 100
        Example:
        2.5(mL) x 10 (kg) +100 = 125 mL/minute
        c. Some neonatal tubing uses a smaller internal diameter requiring calculation of the blood pump speed. Refer to the specific package insert.
        d. The BFR is limited by the vascular access.
    3. Heparin use is determined by specific unit policies. One example might be:
        a. A weight based protocol: Priming dose 20 to 50 units/Kg, followed by continuous drip of Heparin 250 units/mL at 25 units/kg/hr, adjusted to prevent clotting in the dialyzer. (Hansen et al., 2014).
        b. The activated clotting time (ACT) should be > 180 seconds unless bleeding tendencies are a problem. Adjust heparin dose to keep greater than 180 seconds.
        c. Heparin-free dialysis.
            (1) The artificial kidney should be flushed with saline every 20 to 30 minutes throughout run. This volume of fluid must be added to the patient's UF goal and removed during the treatment.
            (2) Monitor the ACT every 20 to 30 minutes.
    4. The estimated dry weight (EDW) needs to be adjusted often since children should be growing and gaining regularly.

E. Preventive care measures.
    1. Immunizations should be current in all children including those with CKD.
    2. Influenza, pneumococcal pneumonia, and hepatitis B vaccinations should be given in addition to all American Academy of Pediatrics (AAP) recommended immunizations (http://www.cispimmunize.org).
    3. Frequent visits for CKD care may make primary care provider (PCP) visits difficult, necessitating vaccinations be offered at the CKD visits.
    4. Rising body mass index (BMI) in children entering ESRD are consistent with the general population and a major concern. In addition, the higher BMI increases the risk for disease progression.

F. Palliative care.
    1. Pediatric palliative care helps children and families live to their fullest potential while facing complex medical conditions.
    2. Care must be child focused, family oriented, and relationship centered.
    3. Care should focus on enhancing quality of life for the child and family while relieving or preventing suffering.

4. Children do not necessarily have the same emotional barriers as adults when talking about death.

5. Discussion may require the help of trained personnel such as child life specialists, psychologists, social workers, psychiatric nurse practitioners, and art therapists, to name a few.

6. It should be an option for parents to make a choice about initiating therapy in a severely disabled child. A child with less disability can do well on kidney replacement therapy, and thus not treating is rarely an option unless a severe disability is present.

SECTION F
Nutrition and Growth

I. Introduction.

A. Pediatric malnutrition is defined as an imbalance between nutrient requirement and intake, resulting in cumulative deficits of energy, protein, or micronutrients that may negatively affect growth. Malnutrition may be illness and/or environmental related and is classified as either acute < 3 months or chronic > 3 months (Mehta et al., 2013).

B. Chronic malnutrition and the impaired growth associated with nutrient imbalances and the inadequate intake of protein-energy are common consequences of CKD (Mehta et al., 2013; Secker, 2013).

C. Regular assessment of the nutritional status and adequacy of nutrient intake are key components in the nutritional management of this high-risk patient population.

D. The focus of nutritional care should be centered around achieving the following overarching goal: To maintain optimal nutrition status and achieve normal growth patterns by ensuring adequate intake of all nutrients and preventing malnutrition, uremic toxicities, and metabolic abnormalities (NKF, 2009b; Secker, 2013).

II. Barriers to achieving goals.

A. Suboptimal energy intake.

B. Anorexia and poor appetite are often associated with taste alterations due to metabolic abnormalities including acidosis, anemia, and uremia.

C. Oral food aversions are common in infants and toddlers, and most young children require supplemental or full enteral nutrition through a feeding tube to meet nutritional goals.

D. Multiple dietary restrictions limit food availability and variety.

E. Cultural influences may make it difficult to meet protein and calorie requirements due to food preferences and religious beliefs.

F Depression, financial concerns, an unstable or stressful living situation, changes in family structure, and fatigue can suppress appetite and intake.

G. Acidosis.

H. Long-term use of corticosteroids to treat kidney disorders and as immunosuppressive therapy posttransplant can impair linear growth.

I. Anemia.

J. Alterations in bone metabolism–mineral bone disorder.

III. Nutritional assessment.

A. Best performed by an experienced pediatric renal dietitian who has received both formal and informal training and education in managing patients with CKD (Secker, 2013).

B Compared with adults, children have variations in their nutritional requirements based on age, stage of CKD, and growth, and they should be assessed on a regular basis (NKF, 2009b).

C. It is suggested that assessments be performed twice as often as that of a healthy child of the same age (NKF, 2009b).

D. Infants and children with polyuria, suboptimal growth parameters, or acute changes in medical status may require more frequent evaluation (NKF, 2009b; Secker, 2013).

E. The nutrition plan should be adjusted frequently depending on response to dietary intervention, growth, biochemical control, changes in medications, medical status, or dialysis modality (KDOQI, 2009; Secker, 2013).

IV. Evaluation of growth/anthropometric measurements. See Table 1.12 for recommended frequency of assessment of children with CKD stages 2 to 5 and 5D and Table 1.13 for criteria for classifying malnutrition.

A. Weight-for-age.
  1. Infants and toddlers 0 to 2 years of age.
    a. Should be undressed and weighed on an infant scale.
    b. Measurements should be taken at least monthly and plotted on the WHO growth charts, recorded to the nearest 0.1 kg.
  2. Children > 2 years old.
    a. Should be weighed with minimal clothing, and without footwear on scales accurate to 100 g.
    b. Measurements should be taken and assessed every 3 to 6 months and plotted on the CDC 2000 growth charts (CDC, 2000).
  3. The fluid status of the patient should be considered when evaluating for weight gain, as positive fluid balance may be falsely interpreted as actual weight gain or increase in lean body mass (LBM) (NKF, 2009b; Secker, 2013).

B. Recumbent length for age/standing height-for-age.
  1. Infants and toddlers 0 to 24 months.
    a. Measured in the supine position on a length board by two people.
    b. One person holds the crown of the head against the head board and the other will move the board up to the infant's heels as the legs are straightened at the knees.
    c. Measurements should be taken at least monthly and plotted on WHO growth charts and recorded to the nearest 0.1 cm.
  2. Children 2 to 20 years.
    a. Standing height for those children that can stand still to get an accurate measurement.
    b. Measurements should be taken and assessed every 3 to 6 months.
    c. Shoes should be removed and measurements plotted on the CDC growth charts and recorded to the nearest 0.1 cm.
  3. Calculation of midparental height to evaluate final growth potential.
    a. Boy – [Paternal Height (cm) + Maternal height (cm) + 13 cm] ÷ 2.
    b. Girl – [Paternal Height (cm) + Maternal height (cm) - 13 cm] ÷ 2.
  4. Head circumference/occipitofrontal circumference (OFC).
    a. Poor head growth is common in children with CKD.
    b. Measure at least monthly in children up to 36 months of age and plot on the head-circumference-for-age growth curve.

Table 1.12

Recommended Frequency of Assessment for Children with CKD stages 2 to 5 and 5D

	Minimum Interval (in months)									
	Age 0 to < 1 year			Age 1–3 year			Age > 3 year			
Measure	CKD 2–3	CKD 4–5	CKD 5D	CKD 2–3	CKD 4–5	CKD 5D	CKD 2	CKD 3	CKD 4–5	CKD 5D
Dietary intake	0.5–3	0.5–3	0.5–2	1–3	1–3	1–3	6–12	6	3–4	3–4
Height or length-for-age percentile or SDS	0.5–1.5	0.5–1.5	0.5–1	1–3	1–2	1	3–6	3–6	1–3	1–3
Height or length velocity-for-age percentile or SDS	0.5–2	0.5–2	0.5–1	1–6	1–3	1–2	6	6	6	6
Estimated dry weight and weight-for-age percentile or SDS	0.5–1.5	0.5–1.5	0.25–1	1–3	1–2	0.5–1	3–6	3–6	1–3	1-3
BMI-for-height-age percentile or SDS	0.5–1.5	0.5–1.5	0.5–1	1–3	1–2	1	3–6	3–6	1–3	1–3
Head circumference-for-age percentile or SDS	0.5–1.5	0.5–1.5	0.5–1	1–3	1–2	1–2	N/A	N/A	N/A	N/A
nPCR	N/A	N/A	N/A	N/A	N/A	N/A	N/A	N/A	N/A	1*

Abbreviation: N/A, not applicable.
*Only applies to adolescents receiving HD.

Adapted from: *American Journal of Kidney Diseases* (2009). *53*(3, Suppl. 2), S16-S26.

Table 1.13

Criteria for Classifying Malnutrition

Measure	Organization	
	Center for Disease Control (CDC)	World Health Organization (WHO)
Underweight	weight/length or BMI < 5th percentile for height age	SDs > -2.0 or BMI < 3rd percentile
Overweight	BMI ≥ 85th percentile for height age	
Obese	BMI > 95th percentile for height age	
Stunting		Length SDs > -2.0 below median
Wasting		Weight SDs > -2.0 below median

Courtesy of Kirsten Thompson.

5. Weight-for-length ratio.
   a. Measures weight relative to height in children 0 to 24 months.
   b. Weight/length < 5th percentile is defined as underweight per the CDC.
6. Body mass index (BMI).
   a. Measures weight relative to height in children 2 to 20 years.
   b. Use BMI for height age (age at which the patient's height is at the 50th percentile) vs. chronological age.
7. BMI < 5th percentile and ≥ 85th percentile for age are associated with increased risk of morbidity and mortality in children with CKD.
8. Other measures. Skinfold thickness measurements such as mid-arm muscle circumference (MAMC), mid-arm circumference (MAC) using calipers, dual x-ray absorptiometry (DEXA), and bio-electrical impedance analysis (BIA) are unreliable methods of estimating body composition in children with CKD as the variance in fluid status affects accuracy and validity.
9. Evaluating growth of preterm infants.
   a. Plot on WHO growth charts for weight and height using corrected age up to 36 months (Mehta et al., 2013).
   b. Plot on Fenton premature growth charts up until 50 weeks corrected age (CDC Growth Charts: 2000).

C. Treating growth failure; indications for growth hormone.
   1. Metabolic abnormalities and nutrient deficiencies

should be identified and aggressively treated in patients whose height or length for age standard deviation score (SDs) is < –2.0 or < 3rd percentile for age prior to starting growth hormone.
2. Correct sodium and fluid losses in patients with polyuria (Secker, 2013).
3. Correct metabolic acidosis. Metabolic acidosis inhibits normal growth. Serum bicarbonate level should be maintained ≥ 22 mmol/L.
4. Recombinant human growth hormone rhGH therapy should be considered if height velocity for age < 3rd percentile persists for > 3 months despite correction of metabolic abnormalities and nutrient deficiencies.
5. Children often achieve catch-up growth and reach adult height within normal time frame for age after long-term growth hormone therapy.

V. Nutritional requirements.

A. Energy – CKD stages 1 to 5, 5D.
   1. Start at the estimated energy requirement (EER) for age for children at a healthy weight (see Tables 1.14 and 1.15).
   2. Energy requirements for kids with CKD are based on those for healthy children given the lack of evidence that suggests increased caloric provision improves growth.
   3. Adjust upward or downward based on growth velocity and weight status.
      a. Malnourished children will likely have higher energy requirements to support "catch-up" growth.
      b. Overweight and obese children often have lower energy requirements. Specialized equations for this population should be used (see Table 1.16).
   4. For children on PD, there is no need to account for dialysate glucose absorption unless overweight or growth velocity exceeds the normal range for age.

B. Protein.
   1. Requirements vary based on age, stage of CKD, and mode of kidney replacement therapy (KRT) (see Table 1.17).
   2. CKD stages 1 to 4.
      a. CKD stages 1 and 2: maintain intake at 100% of the dietary reference intake (DRI) for age at ideal body weight (IBW).
      b. CKD stage 3: maintain daily protein intake (DPI) at 100% to 140% of the DRI for age at IBW.
   3. CKD stage 5 and on dialysis. Patients on dialysis have increased protein requirements to account for losses across the filter and capillary membrane, although the amount is unknown. Losses are higher in PD due to the efficiency of the exchange across the capillary membranes (Secker, 2013; NKF, 2009b).

Table 1.14

Equations to Estimate Energy Requirements for Children at Healthy Weights

Age	Estimated Energy Requirement (EER) (kcal/d) = Total Energy Expenditure + Energy Deposition
0–3 mo	EER = [89 x weight (kg) – 100] + 175
4–6 mo	EER = [89 x weight (kg) – 100] + 56
7–12 mo	EER = [89 x weight (kg) – 100] + 22
13–35 mo	EER = [89 x weight (kg) – 100] + 20
3–8 yr	Boys: EER = 88.5 – 61.9 x age (yr) + PA x [26.7 x weight (kg) + 903 x height (m)] + 20 Girls: EER = 135.3 – 30.8 x age (yr) + PA x [10 x weight (kg) + 934 x height (m)] + 20
9–18 yr	Boys: EER = 88.5 – 61.9 x age (yr) + PA x [26.7 x weight (kg) + 903 x height (m)] + 25 Girls: EER = 135.3 – 30.8 x age (yr) + PA x [10 x weight (kg) + 934 x height (m)] + 25

Source: Health Canada: http://www.hc-sc.gc.ca/fn-an/alt_formats/hpfb-dgpsa/pdf/nutrition/dri_tables-eng.pdf
Reproduced with the permission of the Minister of Public Works and Government Services Canada, 2008.

http://www2.kidney.org/professionals/KDOQI/guidelines_ped_ckd/cpr4.htm

Table 1.15

Physical Activity Coefficients for Determination of Energy Requirements in Children Ages 3 to 18 Years

Gender	Level of Physical Activity			
	Sedentary	Low Active	Active	Very Active
	Typical activities of daily living (ADL) only	ADL + 30–60 min of daily moderate activity (e.g., walking at 5–7 km/h)	ADL + ≥ 60 min of daily moderate activity	ADL + ≥ 60 min of daily moderate activity + an additional 60 min of vigorous activity or 120 min of moderate activity
Boys	1.0	1.13	1.26	1.42
Girls	1.0	1.16	1.31	1.56

Source: Health Canada: http://www.hc-sc.gc.ca/fn-an/alt_formats/hpfb-dgpsa/pdf/nutrition/dri_tables-eng.pdf
Reproduced with the permission of the Minister of Public Works and Government Services Canada, 2008.

http://www2.kidney.org/professionals/KDOQI/guidelines_ped_ckd/cpr4.htm

a. HD: add 0.1g/kg to the DRI for age.
b. PD: add an additional 0.15 to 0.3 g/kg to the DRI for age.
4. The use of high protein oral supplements or modular protein supplements should be considered when children are unable to meet their protein requirements through fluid and food alone (NKF, 2009b).

C. Fluids and electrolytes.
   1. Fluid and sodium.
      a. Sodium is directly linked to fluid balance (Secker, 2013).

b. Fluid intake should be restricted in children who are anuric or oliguric to optimize blood pressure management (NKF, 2009b).
   (1) This can be done by increasing the caloric density of infant formulas either with the formula itself or a modular or using high caloric density ready-to-feed formulas in children and adolescents (see Table 1.18 for a list of formulas and modulars) (Secker, 2013).
   (2) Incremental increases of 2 to 4 calories per ounce may improve tolerance in infants (Secker, 2013).

Table 1.16

Equations to Estimate Energy Requirements for Children Ages 3 to 18 Years Who Are Overweight

Age	Weight Maintenance Total Energy Expenditure (TEE) in Overweight Children
3–18 yr	Boys: TEE = 114 – [50.9 x age (yr)] + PA x [19.5 x weight (kg) + 1161.4 x height (m)]
	Girls: TEE = 389 – [41.2 x age (yr)] + PA x [15.0 x weight (kg) + 701.6 x height (m)]

Source:
http://www2.kidney.org/professionals/KDOQI/guidelines_ped_ckd/cpr4.htm

c. Patients on PD have fewer volume restrictions as they are dialyzed daily (NKF, 2009b).
d. Goal is < 5% interdialytic weight gains (NKF, 2009b).
e. Patients with CKD caused by polyuria.
 (1) They have increased fluid and sodium requirements to account for salt-wasting and high fluid losses.
 (2) They are at risk for impaired growth if losses are not corrected and managed appropriately.
 (3) Sodium supplementation should be considered to maintain normal fluid and sodium balances and promote normal growth.

f. For infants, recommendation to start with 180 to 240 mL/kg of fluid intake per day with 2 to 4 mEq sodium per 100 mL of fluid (Parekh et al., 2001).
g. Sodium supplements should be considered for all infants on PD.
2. Daily sodium intake (NKF, 2009b; Secker, 2013).
 a. Should be restricted to < 1500 mg in patients who have hypertension (i.e., SBP and/or DBP ≥ 95th percentile).
 b. Should be restricted to < 2000 mg in those with prehypertension (i.e., ≥ 90th percentile or < 95th percentile).
3. Potassium.
 a. Hyperkalemia is a common complication of CKD.
 b. Potassium restriction is indicated in patients at risk for hyperkalemia.
 (1) Infants and toddlers: limit to 1 to 3mEq/kg/day.
 (2) Older children and adolescents: limit to 2 to 4 g/day.
 (3) Foods high in potassium such as bananas, chocolate, tomatoes, potatoes, oranges, and avocados should be avoided or limited depending on the degree of hyperkalemia and CKD stage (NKF, 2009b).
 (4) Foods with < 100 mg per serving are considered low in potassium (http://www.kidney.org/atoz/content/foodlabel.cfm).
 (5) Foods with > 200 to 300 mg per serving are

Table 1.17

Recommended Dietary Protein Intake in Children with CKD Stages 3 to 5 and 5D

Age	DRI (g/kg/d)	Recommended for CKD stage 3 (g/kg/d) (100%–140% DRI)	Recommended for CKD stages 4–5 (g/kg/d) (100%–120% DRI)	Recommended for HD (g/kg/d)*	Recommended for PD (g/kg/d) †
0-6 mo	1.5	1.5–2.1	1.5–1.8	1.6	1.8
7-12 mo	1.2	1.2–1.7	1.2–1.5	1.3	1.5
1-3 y	1.05	1.05–1.25	1.05–1.25	1.15	1.3
4-13 y	0.95	0.95–1.15	0.95–1.15	1.05	1.1
14-18 y	0.85	0.85–1.05	0.85–1.05	0.95	1.0

*DRI + 0.1 g/kg/d to compensate for dialytic losses.
†DRI + 0.15-0.3 g/kg/d depending on patient age to compensate for peritoneal losses.

Source: http://www2.kidney.org/professionals/KDOQI/guidelines_ped_ckd/cpr5.htm

considered high in potassium (http://www.kidney.org/atoz/content/foodlabel.cfm.

   c. Hyperkalemia can be treated and prevented by using potassium-reduced infant and adult formulas.

   d. Sodium polystyrene sulfonate (SPS) is a potassium exchange resin that is frequently used to treat hyperkalemia (Bunchman et al., 1991).

     (1) Oral administration is unsafe for neonates and infants given their immature gastrointestinal tracts (Thompson et al., 2013).

     (2) Breast milk and formulas can be treated with SPS prior to administration to avoid oral ingestion. SPS will bind potassium in exchange for sodium leaving a sodium-rich, potassium reduced formula. The formula is decanted leaving a brown precipitate at the bottom (Thompson et al., 2013).

   e. Assess for nondietary sources of hyperkalemia when dietary sources cannot be identified. These may include:

     (1) Metabolic acidosis.

     (2) Inadequate dialysis.

     (3) Medications: tacrolimus, angiotensin-converting enzyme (ACE) inhibitors, and potassium-sparing diuretics.

     (4) Hemolysis.

     (5) Tissue destruction associated with surgery, chemotherapy, or catabolism (Beto & Bansal, 1992).

   f. Potassium restriction is frequently not indicated in patients on PD as they receive daily dialysis (Secker, 2013).

   g. Hypokalemia may be observed in patients on PD and is a common consequence of patients with cystinosis (Secker, 2013).

   h. PD patients receiving daily dialysis frequently require potassium supplementation given the efficiency of capillary exchange (Secker, 2013).

4. Vitamins and minerals.

   a. Provision of 100% DRI for all vitamins (water and fat soluble) and minerals is suggested (IOM, 1997; NKF, 2009b).

   b. Additional supplementation of vitamins and trace elements may be indicated if dietary intake alone does not meet 100% DRI or if there is clinical evidence of deficiency (NFK, 2009b).

   c. An additional water-soluble vitamin (Nephro-Vite tablet or Nephronex liquid) is recommended for children receiving PD or HD therapy to account for losses across the filter (NFK, 2009b).

VI. Evaluating dietary intake.

A. Assessment of dietary history should be performed regularly by a registered dietitian (RD) (refer to Table 1.12) (Secker, 2013).

B. Early identification of food preferences, allergies, and intolerances will help the RD create a meal/eating plan individualized to the child (Secker, 2013).

C. Methods of assessing intake (NKF, 2009b).

   1. 24-hour food recall.

   2. Three-day food record.

   3. Food frequency questionnaire.

   4. iPhone apps.

D. Infants and toddlers.

   1. Healthy infants develop readiness for solids around 4 to 6 months of age (Kleinman, 2009).

   2. Families are instructed and encouraged to follow the same eating and development timeline as that of a healthy child (Secker, 2013).

   3. They frequently show delayed progression through the normal stages of eating (Ravelli, 1995). Common causes may include:

     a. Dislike of solid foods

     b. Fear of varying textures.

     c. Gastroesophageal reflux disease (GERD).

     d. Delayed gastric emptying.

     e. Nausea/emesis.

     f. Altered taste.

     g. Poor appetite.

     h. Constipation and diarrhea.

   4. This makes it difficult for the caregiver to meet the child's nutritional demands through oral intake alone, and a large percentage of children require supplemental feedings (Secker, 2013).

   5. Motility agents, gastric acid suppressants, antimicrobial agents, and probiotics are commonly used to reduce symptoms (Secker, 2013).

E. School-age child (Arts-Rodas & Benoit, 1998; Secker, 2013).

   1. Typically eat independently.

   2. Short stature may invoke teasing by peers and make the child feel self-conscious and worsen self-esteem.

   3. School breakfast and lunch programs may need to be modified to accommodate the child's dietary restrictions.

   4. Include the child in discussions between caregivers and medical staff related to diet, nutrition, growth, laboratory data, and medications.

F. Adolescents (Davis et al., 1996; Secker, 2013).

   1. Peer pressure and the need to assert independence

Table 1.18

Nutrient Composition for Common Formulas and Modulars

NUTRIENTS PER 100 CAL	INFANT FORMULAS					PEDIATRIC FORMULAS								ORAL SUPPLEMENTS	
Formula Type	Breast Milk	Standard Cow's Milk		Semi-Elemental/Allergy		Pediatric Renal Formulas				Standard Formulas		Semi-Elemental		Clear Liquid	
Formula	Breast Milk	Similac PM 60/40	Similac Advance	Nutramigen	Elecare	Suplena	Nepro	Renalcal	Novasource Renal	Pediasure	Boost Kids Essential	Peptamen Jr	Peptamen	Ensure Clear	Boost Breeze
Cal/oz	20	20	20	20	20	53	53	60	60	30	45	30	30	29.4	31.2
kcal/cc	0.67	0.67	0.67	0.67	0.67	1.8	1.8	2	2	1	1.5	1	1	1	1.05
Prot (g)	0.01	2.2	2.1	2.85	3.15	2.5	4.5	1.72	4.5	3	2.8	3	4	3.5	3.6
Fat (g)	5.85	5.7	5.6	5.4	4.8	5.34	5	4.12	4	3.4	5	3.8	3.9	0	0
Ca (mg)	42	56	78	95	116	57	57	3	42	105	97	112	80	0	0
Phos (mg)	21	28	42	52	84	40	40	5	41	84	83	84	70	0	0
Vit A (IU)	338	300	300	300	273	176	176	0	150	211	208	332	430	520	60
Vit D (IU)	3	60	60	50	60	4.7	4.7	0	20	67	56	60	34	25	300
Vit E (IU)	0.6	1.5	1.5	2	2.1	5.4	5.4	0	1.5	2.5	1.5	2.8	3	3.7	24
Vit K (IU)	0.3	8	8	8.1	13	66	66	0	63	23	1.8	20	26	28	2.4
Vit C (mg)	15	9	9	12	9	6	6	3	3	10	606	10	34	10	16
Folate (mcg)	16.5	15	15	16	30	59	59	30	50	25	19	28	54	25	15
B12 (mcg)	0.15	0.25	0.25	0.3	0.4	0.54	0.54	0.3	0.32	0.64	0.16	0.6	0.8	0.5	0.6
Na (mg)	28	24	24	47	45	45	59	3	47	38	46	46	56	17.5	24
Cl (mg)	63	60	65	86	60	52	59	1.5	40	114	49	108	100	18	32
K+ (mg)	80	80	105	110	150	64	59	4	47	131	86	132	150	0	n/a
Fe (mg)	0.09	0.7	1.8	1.8	1.8	1.05	1.05	0	0.9	1.14	0.9	1.4	1.8	1.1	0
Se (mcg)	3	1.8	1.8	2.9	2.6	4.2	4.2	2.5	5.5	3	2.8	3	5	5.2	1.08
Cu (mcg)	45	90	90	75	126	118	118	0	105	84	72	100	200	120	n/a
Zinc (mg)	0.3	0.8	0.75	1	1.15	1.5	1.5	0.7	1.1	0.64	0.56	1.08	2.4	1.5	1.5

Continuation of Table 1.18 from opposite page

MODULARS				
	Benefiber	**Beneprotein**	**Duocal**	**Solcar**
Cals per TBS	15	17	42	23
Protein (g)	0	4	0	0
Fiber (g)	3	0	0	0
Calcium (mg)	0	13	0.425	1.5
Phosphorus (mg)	0	0	0	0.5
Potassium (mg)	10	20	0	0.06
Sodium (mg)	15	10	1.7	4.2

Nutrient Composition for Common Formulas and Modulars courtesy of Kirsten Thompson, MPH, RDN, CSR.

     may inhibit dietary and medication adherence.
2. Irregular eating patterns and meal skipping may compromise the patient's ability to meet nutritional requirements.
3. Should be directly involved in meal planning and diet education.
4. Family members and primary caregivers should be included in discussions to ensure appropriate food is available and encouraged.
5. Families need guidance and ongoing support to establish and reinforce dietary limits.
6. Nutrition education should focus on cafeteria food, fast foods, snacks, and alternative drinks high in sodium and phosphate preservatives.
7. Children and caregivers should be taught how to read ingredient lists and food labels for sodium content and encouraged to limit intake of foods with > 200 mg sodium per serving.
8. Regular physical activity can help reduce catabolism of lean body mass associated with CKD (Montgomery et al., 2006).

VII. Biochemical data.

A. Blood urea nitrogen (BUN).

B. Creatinine.

C. Sodium.

D. Potassium.

E. Carbon Dioxide (CO_2).

F. Chloride.

G. Phosphorus.

H. Calcium.

I. Albumin.

1. Hypoalbuminemia is associated with reduced mortality and morbidity.
2. Hypoalbuminemia is most commonly associated with systemic inflammation and fluid overload, not inadequate protein intake or depleted protein stores.

J. Prealbumin.
1. An acute-phase protein that is degraded by the kidney.
2. Often falsely elevated in patients with CKD.

K. Zinc and copper deficiency may occur in patients on low protein diets and/or with poor intake.

L. Vitamin A and retinol binding protein (RBP).
1. May be a cause of hypercalcemia.
2. RBP is degraded in the kidney.
3. Elevated levels are common as vitamin A and RBP are not removed with dialysis.

M. Normalized Catabolic Rate (nPCR).
1. Used to measure daily protein intake (DPI).
2. Limited to adolescents on HD.
3. Goal: > 1 g/kg/day.

VIII. Nutritional support.

A. Supplemental nutrition may be indicated if the child is unable to meet nutritional demands with usual intake (NKF, 2009b).

B. Specialized formulas with reduced vitamin and mineral content are designed for children with CKD and may be necessary to counteract metabolic imbalances. Refer to Table 1.18 for commonly used infant and pediatric formulas and modulars.

C. Oral nutrition supplements should be trialed first (Secker, 2013).

D. If energy requirements cannot be met, tube feeding with placement of an NG tube for short-term feedings or G-tube for long-term feedings should be considered. Duodenal or jejunal feedings may be indicated in patients with severe reflux or who cannot tolerate gastrostomy enteral feedings (KDOQI, 2009).

E. Feedings can be given as a bolus, as a continuous feeding, or a combination of both.

F. Blenderized tube feedings may be better tolerated in patients with GI disturbances.
1. These feedings are time and labor intensive and may not be appropriate for families or patients with social and financial barriers or for those

patients that require continuous feedings (Novak et al., 2009; Petunik et al., 2001).

2. Recipes can be customized and manipulated to fit the child's fluid, protein, calorie, and micronutrient requirements.

G. Intradialytic parenteral nutrition (IDPN) (NKF, 2009b).
1. The provision of macronutrients (carbohydrates, protein, and fat) through the venous drip chamber of the HD machine.
2. IDPN is intended to supplement enteral intake and should not be viewed as the child's sole source of nutrition.
3. May be indicated for malnourished patients on HD with a BMI for height-age of < 5th percentile who are unable to meet nutritional requirements through oral and tube feedings.
4. Strict criteria must be met in order to justify use of IDPN.
   http://www.kidney.org/professionals/KDOQI/gui delines_ped_ckd/cpr4.htm

H. Intraperitoneal amino acids (IPAA) (Secker, 2013).
1. Substitutes an amino acid solution for one of two glucose exchanges per day when on PD.
2. Routine use is impractical due to high costs and insufficient evidence.
3. May be indicated in patients with malnutrition who have inadequate protein intake.
4. NKF KDOQI guidelines for use should be followed.

SECTION G
Pediatric Pharmacology

I. General considerations for dosing pediatric patients.

A. Drug dosing in pediatric patients.
1. Medications used routinely in pediatric patients do not have pediatric labeling.
   a. There is a lack of safety and efficacy trials in children.
   b. Often used "off-label" based on anecdotal evidence or individual practitioner experience.
2. Adult dose based on body weight in ratio to a pediatric patient's body weight may not be safe or effective.
   a. Children should not be considered small adults.
   b. Higher or lower doses than adult doses may be necessary.
3. During a child's growth and development from

neonate to adolescent, physiologic changes result in varying body composition and organ function as a child ages.
   a. These changes influence drug disposition and the pharmacodynamic response to drugs.
   b. Safe and effective use of drug therapy in pediatric patients requires understanding of the effect of the child's stage of development on the properties of the drug.
4. Neonates, especially premature neonates, have the most variable body composition and organ function of any pediatric population.

B. Pharmacokinetic differences.
1. Absorption.
   a. During growth from a neonate to an adult, many gastrointestinal tract factors related to oral absorption undergo significant maturational changes.
      (1) Infants under 6 to 8 months of age have delayed gastric emptying, so may have decreased rate of drug absorption and/or increased bioavailability due to slow intestinal transit.
      (2) Alterations in pancreatic enzymes and bile salt production may also increase the bioavailability of drugs in infants or alter their absorption.
      (3) In children and infants less than 2 years of age, bacterial colonization of the intestines may also cause changes in drug bioavailability.
   b. Neonates, in particular those who are premature, have variable intramuscular absorption.
   c. Percutaneous absorption is increased in pediatric patients due to a variety of factors.
   d. Topical drugs should be used cautiously in premature neonates. Absorption is particularly pronounced in these patients and may result in toxic effects.
2. Distribution.
   a. Distribution differences in children vs. adults are caused by relative proportions of body water and fat and differences in protein binding.
   b. Total body water is highest in premature newborns and approaches adult values by early adolescence. Drugs that distribute into extracellular fluid will have higher volumes of distribution in smaller children, so may require larger milligram-per-kilogram doses to achieve similar concentrations.
   c. Total body fat varies based on age and has fluctuations from infancy throughout childhood and adolescence. Due to their higher percentage of body fat, neonates and infants

will have a higher volume of distribution for lipophilic drugs.

   d. Caution should be used in drug dosing in obese patients of any age.

     (1) Obesity will increase volume of distribution for lipophilic drugs, requiring higher doses.

     (2) May cause overdoses if actual body weight is used in calculating doses of hydrophilic drugs due to lower percentage of extracellular water in obesity.

   e. Since the pharmacologic action of drugs is that of the free (unbound) portion of the drug, alterations in protein binding can lead to alterations in drug effect and/or possible toxicity. Protein binding is less in neonates and approaches adult values by the first year of life.

3. Metabolism.

   a. Most drug metabolism occurs in the liver.

   b. Liver enzyme activity is greatly dependent on patient age. Different enzymes follow different patterns of development of maturity from infancy to adulthood.

4. Elimination.

   a. Most drugs (or their metabolites) are excreted through the kidneys.

   b. Overall functional capacity of the kidney increases with age up to early adulthood.

   c. As kidney function decreases, doses should be adjusted based on kidney function to avoid drug toxicity.

C. Medication administration.

1. Safe dose ranges should be determined according to both the child's age and weight, and/or body surface area (BSA).

2. For painful routes of administration, and also for some routes of administration, such as otic or optic, which are not painful but may be uncomfortable or unpleasant to children, involving trusted caregivers in administration is important. Play, patience, and calming techniques are helpful.

3. Routes of administration.

   a. Oral.

     (1) If liquid dosage forms are not readily available, seek advice from a pharmacist as to whether crushing or splitting tablets or opening capsules is appropriate.

     (2) Measure oral liquids with an oral syringe or medicine cup at eye level.

       (a) If possible, administer medications to infants while on a parent's lap in a semi-reclining position.

       (b) Give medication slowly in the side of the mouth.

       (c) Allow toddlers to participate and take medications independently if possible.

       (d) Involve parents and use positive reinforcement and praise.

       (e) Do not disguise medications in a drink or bottle.

     (3) School-age children may begin learning pill-swallowing techniques but may require encouragement and extra time until the skill is mastered.

     (4) Observe teenage patients to ensure medications are consumed.

   b. Nasogastric, orogastric, or gastrostomy tubes.

     (1) Avoid the use of tablets if possible.

     (2) If liquid dosage forms are not readily available, seek advice from a pharmacist as to whether crushing or splitting tablets or opening capsules is appropriate.

     (3) If crushing tablets, crush to a fine powder and mix with sterile water.

     (4) Flush the tube with water between medications and following use with an appropriate volume to the size of the tube.

   c. Intramuscular.

     (1) The vastus lateralis muscle is the traditional site for injections in newborns, infants, and small children.

     (2) Use caution when using the deltoid muscle for injections in children less than 5 years of age.

     (3) The gluteus maximus muscle is not generally recommended as an injection site in children.

     (4) A maximum injection volume of 1 mL, particularly in children under 2 years old, is recommended.

   d. Rectal.

     (1) Use side lying position. With infants, it is possible to lift the legs and flex the knees, as while changing a diaper.

     (2) Insert a lubricated suppository up to the first knuckle.

     (3) Hold the buttocks together for several minutes.

     (4) Do not cut or divide suppositories.

II. Medications specific to children.

A. Growth hormone.

1. Should be started for patients with growth failure and continued until the time of transplant.

2. Subcutaneous injection preferred; can be given IM.

3. Do not shake vial.

4. Rotate injection sites in the thigh, buttock, or abdomen.

5. If patient is on hemodialysis, give at night 3 to 4 hours after dialysis.

6. If patient is on chronic cyclic peritoneal dialysis, give in the morning after dialysis.
7. If patient is on chronic ambulatory peritoneal dialysis, give at night at the time of overnight exchange.

B. Childhood immunization schedule.
   1. Routine immunizations should be kept as current as possible throughout the stages of kidney disease.
   2. Immune response to vaccines may decline as kidney function declines.
   3. Live vaccines cannot be given posttransplant.

III. Differences in medications when used in pediatric patients.

A. CKD and dialysis.
   1. Analgesics.
      a. Children are more susceptible to respiratory depression caused by narcotics, particularly infants less than 3 months of age and those who are premature.
      b. Lower doses of narcotic doses are recommended in infants vs. older children and should be titrated to effect.
      c. Never alter a narcotic patch or controlled or extended-release tablet or patch to make it suitable for administration to a child by crushing, breaking, or cutting the product. Choose an alternate dosage form.
      d. When gabapentin is used for seizures or analgesia, children are more likely than adults to experience behavior issues such as emotional lability and hostility.
   2. Antacids.
      a. Chilling sodium citrate solution increases palatability.
      b. Sodium bicarbonate tablets may be crushed if sodium citrate solution is not tolerated.
   3. Antianemics.
      a. Accidental iron overdose.
         (1) A leading cause of fatal poisoning in children under the age of 6.
         (2) Instruct families to store oral iron preparations out of children's reach and in child-resistant containers and to follow dosing instructions carefully.
         (3) Immediate care should be sought in the case of accidental overdose.
      b. Consider all sources of iron intake when evaluating oral iron doses to avoid overdose, including iron provided by infant or enteral formulas and nutritional supplements.
      c. Multiple concentrations of liquid oral iron supplements exist. Careful attention must be paid to the elemental iron content when

administering iron to avoid incorrect substitution of one liquid concentration for another and the potential for serious over or under-dosing.
      d. Do not administer oral iron with milk or milk-based infant or enteral formulas.
      e. Liquid oral iron products may cause staining of the teeth, but this can usually be reversed.
   4. Antidiarrheals.
      a. Loperamide.
         (1) Avoid use in infants and children, particularly those younger than 3 years of age, with acute diarrhea due to serious risk of adverse events and possible death.
         (2) The manufacturer does not recommend use of loperamide in children less than 2 years of age.
         (3) However, dosing recommendations for children as young as 2 months of age with chronic diarrhea due to noninfectious causes are available.
      b. Diphenoxylate/atropine should be used with caution in children.
         (1) The lowest effective dose should be used.
         (2) Even at recommended doses, atropinism (dehydration, tachycardia, urinary retention) may develop.
         (3) Overdosage may result in severe respiratory depression, coma, or permanent brain damage.
         (4) Do not use in children under the age of .
         (5) Measure doses carefully.
   5. Antiemetics.
      a. Phenothiazines.
         (1) Have a high incidence of extrapyramidal reactions and episodes of respiratory depression in children.
         (2) Their use, particularly in children less than 5 years of age, should be limited to patients who do not respond to other antiemetics.
         (3) The lowest effective dose should be used with extreme caution.
         (4) Phenothiazines should never be used in patients who are less than 2 years of age or weigh less than 9 kg due to the potential for severe and possibly fatal respiratory depression.
      b. Droperidol should only be used in children who do not respond to other antiemetics.
      c. For children who cannot swallow tablets, the injection form of dolasetron can be given orally by mixing it in apple or apple-grape juice, or a pharmacist can compound an oral suspension using the tablets.
   6. Antilipemics.
      a. Limited dosing data is available for antilipemics

in children less than 8 years of age, with no dosing available for fibric acid derivatives.

b. Bile-sequestering agents are available as powders or granules for administration in liquid.
   (1) However, HMG CoA reductase inhibitors are only available in tablet formulations.
   (2) Some tablet formulations can be cut or crushed.

c. More frequent laboratory monitoring for adverse events, such as liver dysfunction associated with HMG CoA reductase inhibitors, is recommended for children vs. adults.

7. Antihypertensives.
   a. Pediatric dosing recommendations are available for at least one medication in all classes of antihypertensives commonly used in CKD and patients on dialysis.
   b. Few antihypertensives are commercially available in oral liquid dosage forms suitable for young children. But pharmacists can compound oral solutions for many commonly used medications, such as amlodipine, atenolol, clonidine, isradipine, labetalol, and lisinopril.

8. Antimicrobials.
   a. Tetracyclines should not be given to children less than 8 years old due to permanent discoloration of teeth and retardation of skeletal development and bone growth.
   b. Fluroquinolones are not a drug of first choice in children due to incidence of adverse events related to joints and the surrounding tissues.

9. Cardiotonics.
   a. With excessive dosing, children are more likely to experience cardiac arrhythmia.
   b. Infants may have bradycardia as a sign of digoxin toxicity.
   c. Any arrhythmia in a child on digoxin should be considered a sign of toxicity.

10. Glucocorticoids.
    a. The risk of hypothalamic-pituitary-adrenal (HPA) suppression is higher in children, particularly young children.
       (1) Acute adrenal insufficiency may occur with abrupt withdrawal after long-term therapy or with stress.
       (2) Taper doses slowly and consider additional doses prior to and during unusual stress, such as surgery.
    b. May cause osteoporosis or inhibition of bone grown and reduction of growth velocity in children. Monitor growth and bone development.
    c. Oral palatability can be problematic. Prednisolone sodium phosphate is the most palatable vs. other formulations. Chilling the solution further improves tolerability.

11. Proton pump inhibitors.

a. Omeprazole capsules may be opened and sprinkled on applesauce. Powder packets for oral suspension or a pharmacist-prepared oral solution may be used for nasogastric tube administration.

b. Lansoprazole oral solution may also be compounded by a pharmacist.
   (1) Capsules may be opened and sprinkled on soft food such as pudding or applesauce or mixed in approximately 60 mL of apple, orange, or tomato juice.
   (2) The drug may be given via nasogastric tube by mixing (not crushing) with apple juice.

c. Orally-disintegrating tablets may be dissolved in water and given orally or via nasogastric tube.

12. Sedative-hypnotics. There is very limited data available on effectiveness or dosing of sedative-hypnotics in children.

B. Transplantation.
   1. Immunosuppressive medications.
      a. Tacrolimus.
         (1) Compared to older children, adolescents, or adults, younger children generally require higher maintenance doses of tacrolimus on a mg/kg basis – approximately two times higher.
         (2) Tacrolimus may be compounded to suspension by a pharmacist.
         (3) Different preparations exist; verify concentrations to avoid dosing errors.
      b. Cyclosporine.
         (1) The oral solution form can be mixed with room temperature milk or orange or apple juice to improve palatability.
         (2) Do allow to stand in milk – stir and have the patient drink immediately.
      c. Everolimus tablets and tablets for oral suspension are not interchangeable. Oral tablets can be dispersed in water.
      d. Mycophenolate mofetil tablets, capsules, and suspension are not interchangeable with delayed-release tablets.
      e. Azathioprine may be compounded to an oral suspension by a pharmacist.
      f. Sirolimus may inhibit skeletal and muscle growth. Monitor the patient for growth failure.
   2. Antivirals.
      a. Dosing information and dosage forms for pediatric patients is not available for famciclovir.
      b. Valacyclovir tablets can be compounded into a suspension for oral use by a pharmacist.
   3. Antifungals. For young children who cannot swish nystatin about the mouth or retain it in the mouth, it can be painted into the recesses of the mouth with a cotton swab.

4. Phosphorous supplements.
   a. Due to confusion with milliequivalents vs. millimoles, the most reliable method of dosing phosphorous is in mmol.
   b. Phosphorous provided from dietary intake should be considered in calculating the total daily dose.
   c. Phosphorous will be provided in either a potassium or sodium salt form, depending on the product chosen. The amount of potassium and/or sodium provided in the product should also be considered in light of the patient's laboratory values.

IV. Psychosocial issues.

A. The impact of kidney disease on the child and family changes family dynamics.
   1. Care for a child with a chronic illness involves considerable psychological and social stress.
   2. Autonomy development.
      a. Requires attention to issues of overprotection by parents or caregivers of the chronically ill child.
      b. This is made especially difficult if the parent is the caregiver "controlling" the dialysis treatments.
      c. The overprotection often is a misguided attempt to compensate for the child's "suffering."
   3. Parents and/or caregivers need help in understanding how to discipline and what expectations to set for the child.
   4. Respite for the caregivers is to be encouraged when possible to help avoid burnout and depression.

B. Nursing care.
   1. Parents and caregivers need anticipatory guidance in developing expectations for the child (refer to Table 1.1, Developmental Age-Appropriate Care: Preparation/Education/Activity).
   2. Social development and self-esteem requires peer relationships.
   3. Adolescents may need support for dealing with rejection for being different at a time when conformity determines body image and identity.
   4. Adolescents may need strategies for developing close relationships with peers to assist in development of body image, self-esteem, and independence.
   5. Transition from childhood to adulthood is a key mediating role for adult quality of life.
   6. Help with the transition into adult life from family life to independent life and from school to employment.
   7. School completion will assist in the transition and set expectations for an adult life.

C. Methods to promote adherence to treatment.
   1. Factors that may influence patient's adherence to therapy and/or medication regimen.
      a. Misunderstanding of therapy or medication dose changes.
      b. Belief that therapy and/or medications are not helpful.
      c. Disorganized family structure.
      d. Adolescence.
      e. Complexity of therapy and/or medication regimen.
      f. Body image changes.
   2. Factors that help adherence.
      a. Simplification of therapy and/or medication administration and dosage times.
      b. Ongoing education.
      c. Frequent clinic visits.
      d. Behavior modification.
      e. Involvement of adolescents in self-care to promote independence.
      f. Planning for a future and developing life goals.
      g. Counseling must be individualized and/or family based.

D. Providing pediatric care.
   1. Partner with patients and families as members of the healthcare team.
   2. Treat each family with dignity and respect.
      a. Listen to patient and family perspectives and choices.
      b. Incorporate patient and family knowledge, values, beliefs, and cultural backgrounds into care planning and delivery.
   3. Build partnerships based on mutual respect and open communication.
      a. Respect each family's uniqueness.
      b. Listen carefully to understand perspectives and needs of families.
   4. Share information clearly, completely, and consistently.
      a. Communicate and share information with each patient and family in ways that are affirming and useful.
      b. Ensure privacy and confidentiality.
      c. Respond flexibly to the family's needs, and negotiate differences of opinion in a timely and respectful manner.
      d. Promote and value competency and expertise each member brings to the healthcare team.
      e. Include providers/services in family's home, community, and school in the care team.
      f. Allow patient/family's participation in decision making and care planning by assuring timely, complete, accurate information.

E. Patient and family education.
   1. Children with CKD need special attention paid to

learning and developing skills for social and independent functioning.

2. Achieving age-specific developmental milestones is important in adjustment to adult life.

3. Whenever appropriate, children should be included in planning, implementing, and taking responsibility for their own care.

4. Education of parent and caregiver should be done at the 5th to 6th grade reading level.

5. The parent and caregiver may need assessment for ability to read or other cognitive dysfunction.

6. Parents need written materials for training as well as visual and verbal cues.

7. Monthly clinic visits are opportunities to teach and reinforce prior teaching.

F. The pediatric patient in an adult unit.
   1. An adult unit must have the resources, both staff and equipment, to meet the safety needs of the pediatric patient.
      a. Pediatric patients are not just little adults. They respond differently and can be challenging.
      b. Maintaining fluid balance is a major concern.
      c. Patients must achieve dry weight or risk serious complications from LVH, chronic fluid overload, and potential cardiac complications.
      d. Crying and manipulative behaviors may hinder the staff in the process of fluid removal.
   2. Transition to adult care.
      a. Transition from childhood to adulthood plays a key mediating role for later quality of life.
      b. Chronic illness may complicate the transition into adult life.
         (1) From family to independent life.
         (2) From school to employment.
      c. Transition programs should place expectations on the child.
      d. Independence requires that the child knows his/her medications, dialysis therapy parameters, health history, diet, and the significance of relating to care providers.
      e. Adult care providers will expect that the child will be able to manage his/her own appointments; the child needs to be prepared to assume that responsibility.

References

Alliance for Paired Donation (2009). *Main page.* Retrieved from http://www.paireddonation.org/

Alparslan, C., Yavascan, O., Bal, A., Kanik, A., Kose, E., Demir, B.K., & Aksu, N. (2012). The performance of acute peritoneal dialysis treatment in neonatal period. *Renal Failure, 34*(8), 1015-1020. doi:10.3109/0886022X.2012.708378

Andreoli, S.P., Brewer, E.D., Watkins, S., Fivush, B., Powe, N., Shevchek, J., & Foreman, J. (2005). American Society of Pediatric Nephrology position paper on linking reimbursement to quality of care. *Journal of the American Society of Nephrologists, 16,* 2263-2269. doi: 10.1681/ASN.2005020186

Arts-Rodas, D., & Benoit, D (1998). Feeding problems in infancy and early childhood: Identification and management. *Paediatrics & Child Health, 3,* 21-27.

Askenazi, D.J., Goldstein, S.L., Koralkar, R., Fortenberry, J., Baum, M., Hackbarth, R., ... Somers, M.J. (2013). Continuous renal replacement therapy for children < =10 kg: A report from the prospective pediatric continuous renal replacement therapy registry. *Journal of Pediatrics, 162*(3), 587-592 e583. doi:10.1016/j.jpeds.2012.08.044

Askenazi, D. J., Griffin, R., McGwin, G., Carlo, W., & Ambalavanan, N (2009). Acute kidney injury is independently associated with mortality in very low birthweight infants: A matched case-control analysis. *Pediatric Nephrology, 24*(5), 991-997. doi:10.1007/s00467-009-1133-x

Askenazi, D.J., Feig, D.I., Graham, N.M., Hui-Stickle, S., & Goldstein, S. L. (2006). 3–5 year longitudinal follow-up of pediatric patients after acute renal failure. *Kidney International, 69*(1), 184-189. doi:10.1038/sj.ki.5000032

Avery, R.K., & Michaels, M. (2008). Update on immunizations in solid organ transplant recipients: What clinicians need to know. American *Journal of Transplantation, 8*(1), 9-14.

Bauer, P., Reinhart, K., & Bauer, M. (2008). Significance of venous oximetry in the critically ill. *MedIntensiva, 32*(30), 134-142.

Beck, L., Bomback, A.S., Choi, M.J., Holzman, L.B., Langford,C., Mariani, L.H., ... Waldman, M. (2013). KDOQI US commentary on the 2012 KDIGO clinical practice guideline for glomerulonephritis. *American Journal of Kidney Diseases, 62*(3), 403-441.

Beto, J., & Bansal, V.K. (1992). Hyperkalemia: Evaluating dietary and nondietary etiology. *Journal of Renal Nutrition, 2,* 28-29.

Boyle, A., & Sobotka, P.A. (2006). Redefining the therapeutic objective in decompensated heart failure: Hemoconcentration as a surrogate for plasma refill rate. *Journal of Cardiac Failure, 12*(4), 246-249.

Brophy, P.D., Mottes, T.A., Kudelka, T.L., McBryde, K.D., Gardner, J.J., Maxvold, N.J., & Bunchman, T.E. (2001). AN-69 membrane reactions are pH-dependent and preventable. *American Journal of Kidney Diseases, 38*(1), 173-178. doi:10.1053/ajkd.2001.25212

Bunchman, T.E., Wood, E.G., Schenck, M.H., Weaver, K.A., Klein, B.L., & Lynch, R.E. (1991). Pretreatment of formula with sodium polystyrene sulfonate to reduce dietary potassium intake. *Pediatric Nephrology, 5,* 29-32.

Bunchman, T.E., Brophy, P.D., & Goldstein, S.L. (2008). Technical considerations for renal replacement therapy in children. *Seminars in Nephrology, 28*(5), 488-492. doi:10.1016/j.semnephrol.2008.05.009

Centers for Disease Control and Prevention (CDC) (2000). Use and interpretation of the CDC growth charts. Retrieved from http://www.cdc.gov/growthcharts/2000growthchart-us.pdf

Chand, D.H., & Valentini, R.P (2008). International pediatric fistula first initiative: A call to action. *American Journal of Kidney Diseases, 51,* 1016-1024.

Chand, D.H., Valentini, R.P., & Kamil, E.S. (2009). Hemodialysis vascular access options in pediatrics: Considerations for patients and practitioners. *Pediatric Nephrology, 24,* 1121-1128.

Chavers, B.M., Solid, C.A., Gilbertson, D.T., & Collins, A.J. (2007). Infection-related hospitalization rates in pediatric versus adult patients with end-stage renal disease in the United States. *Journal of the American Society of Nephrology, 18,* 952-959. doi:10.1681/ASN.2006040406

Cordtz, J., Olde, B., Solem, K., & Ladefoged, S.D. (2008). Central venous oxygen saturation and thoracic admittance during dialysis: New approaches to hemodynamic monitoring. *Hemodialysis International 12*(3), 369-377.

Counts, C. (Ed.). (2008). *Core curriculum for nephrology nurses* (5th ed.). Pitman, NJ: American Nephrology Nurses Association.

Cupples, S.A., & Ohler, L. (Eds.). (2008). *Core curriculum for transplant nurses.* St. Louis: Mosby Elsevier.

Davis, M.C., Tucker, C.M., & Fennell, R.S. (1996). Family behavior, adaptation, and treatment adherence of pediatric nephrology patients. *Pediatric Nephrology, 6,*198-194.

Devuyst, O., Konrad, M., Jeunemaitre, Z., & Zennaro, M. (2009). Tubular disorders of electrolyte regulation. In E.D. Avner, W.E. Harmon, P. Niaudet, & N. Yoshikawa (Eds.), *Pediatric nephrology* (6th ed., pp 929-977). Berlin Heidelberg: Springer-Verlag.

Diroll, A. (2011). Blood volume monitoring a crucial step in reducing mortality. *Nephrology News & Issues, 25*(2), 32.

Fadrowski, J.J., Hwang, W., Frankenfield, D.L., Fivush, B.A., Neu, A.M., & Furth, S.L. (2006). Clinical course associated with vascular access type in a national cohort of adolescents who receive hemodialysis: Findings from the clinical performance measures and U.S. renal data system projects. *Clinical Journal of the American Society of Nephrology, 1,* 987-992.

Flynn, J. (2013). Hypertension is difficult to control in children, too. *American Journal of Hypertension, 26*(7), 841-842.

Flynn, J. (2011). Obesity hypertension in adolescents: Epidemiology, evaluation, and management obesity hypertension in adolescents. *The Journal of Clinical Hypertension, 13*(5), p. 323. doi:10.1111/j.1751-7176.2011.00452.x

Gahl, W. (2009). Cystinosis. In E.D. Avner, W.E. Harmon, P. Niaudet, & N. Yoshikawa (Eds.), *Pediatric nephrology* (6th ed., pp. 1017-1038). Berlin Heidelberg: Springer-Verlag.

Gadegbeku, C.A., Gipson, D.S., Holzman, L.B., Ojo, A.O., Song, P., Barisoni, L., … Kretzler, M. (2013). Design of the Nephrotic Syndrome Study Network (NEPTUNE) to evaluate primary glomerular nephropathy by a multidisciplinary approach. *Kidney International, 83*(4), 749-756. doi:10.1038/ki.2012.428

Gipson, D.S., Massengill, S.F., Yao, L., Nagaraj, S., Smoyer, W.E., Mahan, J.D., … Greenbaum, L.A. (2014) Management of childhood onset nephrotic syndrome. *Pediatrics, 124*(2), 747. Originally published online July 27, 2009. doi:10.1542/peds.2008-1559

Hackbarth, R., Bunchman, T.E., Chua, A.N., Somers, M.J., Baum, M., Symons, J. M., . . . Goldstein, S.L. (2007). The effect of vascular access location and size on circuit survival in pediatric continuous renal replacement therapy: A report from the PPCRRT registry. *International Journal of Artificial Organs, 30*(12), 1116-1121.

Hansen, C., McAfee, N., & Munshi, R. (2014). Standardized heparin dosing in pediatric dialysis unit. *Hemodialysis International, 18*(1), 226-227.

Hogg, R.J., Furth, S., Lemley, K.V., Portman, R., Schwartz, G.W., Coresh, J., … Levey, A.S. (2003). National Kidney Foundation's Kidney Disease Outcomes Quality Initiative clinical practice guidelines for chronic kidney disease in children and adolescents: Evaluation, classification, and stratification. *Pediatrics, 111,* 1416-1421.

Honda, M., & Warady, B.A. (2010). Long-term peritoneal dialysis and encapsulating peritoneal sclerosis in children. *Pediatric Nephrology, 25*(1), 75-81. doi:10.1007/s00467-008-0982-z

Igarashi, T. (2009). Fanconi syndrome. In E.D. Avner, W.E. Harmon, P. Niaudet, & N. Yoshikawa (Eds.), *Pediatric nephrology* (6th ed., pp. 1040-1067). Berlin Heidelberg: Springer-Verlag.

Institute of Medicine (IOM). (1997). Dietary reference intakes for calcium, phosphorus, magnesium, vitamin D and fluoride. Washington, DC: National Academies Press.

Kerlin, B.A., Ayoob, R., & Smoyer, W.E. (2012). *Clinical Journal of the American Society of Nephrology, 7*(3), 513–520. doi:10.2215/CJN.10131011

Kidney Disease: Improving Global Outcomes (KDIGO). (2012a). KDIGO Clinical practice guideline for acute kidney injury. *Kidney International Supplements, 2*(1), 1-138. doi:10.1038/kisup.2012.1

Kidney Disease: Improving Global Outcomes (KDIGO). (2012b). Glomerulonephritis Work Group. KDIGO clinical practice guideline for glomerulonephritis. *Kidney International Supplement, 2,* 139–274.

Kleinman, R.E. (2009). Committee on Nutrition. *Pediatric nutrition handbook* (p. 1470). Elk Grove Village, IL: American Academy of Pediatrics.

Kong, X., Yuan, H., Fan, J., Li, Z., Wu, T., & Jiang, L. (2013). Lipid-lowering agents for nephrotic syndrome. *Cochrane Database of Systematic Reviews.* doi:10.1002/14651858

Ma, A., Shroff, R., Hothi, D., Lopez, M.M., Veligratli, F., Calder, F., & Rees, L. (2013). A comparison of arteriovenous fistulas and central venous lines for long-term chronic hemodialysis. *Pediatric Nephrology, 28*(2), 321-326. doi:10.1007/s00467-012-2318-2

Mak, R.H., & Warady, B.A. (2013). Dialysis: Vascular access in children – Arteriovenous or CVC? *Nature Reviews Nephrology, 9*(1), 9-11. doi:10.1038/nrneph.2012.265

Mammen, C., Al Abbas, A., Skippen, P., Nadel, H., Levine, D., Collet, J.P., & Matsell, D.G (2012). Long-term risk of CKD in children surviving episodes of acute kidney injury in the intensive care unit: A prospective cohort study. *American Journal of Kidney Diseases, 59*(4), 523-530. doi:10.1053/j.ajkd.2011.10.048

Manook, M., & Calder, F. (2012). Practical aspect of arteriovenous fistula formation in the pediatric population. *Pediatric Nephrology, 28,* 885-893.

McCarthy, J.H., & Tizard, E.J. (2010). Clinical practice: Diagnosis and management of Henoch-Schönlein purpura. *European Journal of Pediatrics, 169*(6), 643-650.

Mehta, N.M., Corkins, M.R., Lyman, B., Malone, A., Goday, P.S., Carney, L.N. … Schwenk, W.F. (2013). Defining pediatric malnutrition: A paradigm shift toward etiology-related definitions. *Journal of Parenteral and Enteral Nutrition, 37*(4), 460-81. doi: 10.1177/0148607113479972

Michael, M., Brewer, E.D., & Goldstein, S.L. (2004). Blood volume monitoring to achieve target weight in pediatric hemodialysis patients. *Pediatric Nephrology, 19*(4), 432-437. doi:10.1007/s00467-003-1400-1

Montgomery, L., Parker, T., MacDougall, K., & Goldstein, S. (2006). Effect of twice weekly exercise for pediatric hemodialysis patients. *Hemodialysis International, 10,* 129-130.

National Institutes of Health (NIH). (2004). National Heart, Lung, and Blood Institute: The fourth report on the diagnosis, evaluation, and treatment of high blood pressure in children and adolescents. *Pediatrics, 114*(2), 555-576.

National Kidney Foundation Kidney Disease Outcomes Quality Initiative (NKF KDOQI). (2002). Part 7. Stratification of risk for progression of kidney disease and development of cardiovascular disease (pp. 197-249). *KDOQI Clinical Practice Guidelines for Chronic Kidney Disease.* New York: Author.

National Kidney Foundation (NFK). (2002). K/DOQI clinical practice guidelines for chronic kidney disease: Evaluation, classification, and stratification. *American Journal of Kidney Diseases, 39*(2)(Suppl. 1), S1-266.

National Kidney Foundation (NFK). (2006a). KDOQI clinical practice guidelines and clinical practice guidelines on hypertension and antihypertensive agents in chronic kidney disease. *American Journal of Kidney Diseases, 48*(Suppl. 1), S2-90.

National Kidney Foundation (NFK). (2006b). KDOQI clinical practice guidelines for vascular access: update 2006. *American Journal of Kidney Diseases, 348*(Suppl. 1), S227–S409.

National Kidney Foundation. (2009a). *Your guide to the new food label.* Retrieved from http://www.kidney.org/atoz/content/foodlabel.cfm.

National Kidney Foundation. (2009b). KDOQI clinical practice guideline for nutrition in children with CKD: 2008 update. *American Journal of Kidney Diseases, 53*(Suppl. 2), S1-S124.

North American Pediatric Clinical Trials and Collaborative Studies (NAPRTCS). (2010). *2010 Annual Report* (p. 11). Retrieved October 7, 2013, from https://web.emmes.com/study/ped/annlrept/2010_Report.pdf

North American Pediatric Renal Trials and Collaborative Studies (NAPRTCS). (2011). *NAPRTCS 2011 annual dialysis report.* Retrieved from https://emmes.com/study/ped/annlrept/annualrept2011.pdf

Novak, P., Wilson, K., Ausderau, K., & Cullinane, D. (2009). The use of blenderized tube feedings. Infant, *Child, & Adolescent Nutrition (ICAN), 1*(1), 21-23. doi:10.1177/1941406408329196

Organ Procurement and Transplantation Network (OPTN) and Scientific Registry of Transplant Recipients (SRTR). (2011). *OPTN/SRTR 2011 annual data report.* Department of Health and Human Services, Health Resources and Services Administration, Healthcare Systems Bureau, Division of Transplantation. Retrieved from http://srtr.transplant.hrsa.gov/annual_reports/2011/pdf/pp/01_kidney12.zip

Organ Procurement and Transplantation Network (OPTN). (2012). Department of Health and Human Services, Health Resources and Services Administration, Healthcare Systems Bureau, Division of Transplantation. Retrieved October 8, 2013 from http://optn.transplant.hrsa.gov/resources/allocationcalculators.asp?index=78

Parekh, R.S., Flynn, J.T., Smoyer, W.E., Milne, J.L., Kershaw, D.B., Bunchman, T.E., & Sedman, A.B. (2002). Improved growth in young children with severe chronic renal insufficiency who use specified nutritional therapy. *Journal of the American Society of Nephrology, 13*(5), 1421-1422.

Patel, H.P., Goldstein, S.L., Mahan, J.D., Smith, B., Fried, C.B., Currier, H., & Flynn, J.T. (2007). Improved BP control using noninvasive monitoring of hematocrit. *Clinical Journal of the American Society of Nephrology, 2*, 252-257.

Petunik, S., O'Flaherty, T., Santoro, K., Willging, P., & Kaul, A. (2001). Pureed by gastrostomy tube diet improves gagging and retching in children with fundoplication. *Journal of Parenteral and Enteral Nutrition, 35*, 375.

Ponticelli, C., Moia, M., & Montagnino, G. (2009). Renal allograft thrombosis. *Nephrology Dialysis Transplantation, 24*(5), 1388-1393.

Ravelli, A.M. (1995). Gastrointestinal function in chronic renal failure. *Pediatric Nephrology, 9*, 756-762.

Reyes-Bahamonde, J., Raimann, J.G., Thijssen, S., Levin N.W., & Kotanko, P. (2013). Fluid overload and inflammation – A vicious cycle. *Seminars in Dialysis, 26*(1), 31-35. doi:10.1111/sdi.12024

Richardson, M.A. (2012). Epidemiology and pathophysiology of nephrotic syndrome-associated thromboembolic disease (Quiz 375). *Nephrology Nursing Journal, 39*(5), 365-374. quiz 375.

Rodriguez, H., Domenici, R., Diroll, A., & Goykhman, L. (2005). Assessment of dry weight by monitoring changes in blood volume during hemodialysis using Crit-Line. *Kidney International, 68*(2), 854–861.

Sayed, B., Amaral, S., Kutner, N., & Patzer, R (2013). Survival benefits of preemptive renal transplantation for pediatric end stage renal disease patients. *2013 ATC Abstracts.* Retrieved October 7, 2013, from http://www.atcmeetingabstracts.com/abstract/survival-benefits-of-preemptive-renal-transplantation-for-pediatric-end-stage-renal-disease-patients/

Schmitt, C.P., & Mehis, O. (2011). Mineral and bone disorders in children with chronic kidney disease. *Nature Reviews Nephrology, 7*(11), 624.

Schwartz, G.J., & Work, D.F. (2009). Measurement and estimation of GFR in children and adolescents. *Clinical Journal of the American Society of Nephrology, 4*, 1832-1843.

Secker, D. (2013). Nutrition management of chronic kidney disease in the pediatric patient. In L. Byham-Gray, J. Stover, & K. Wiesen (Eds.), *A Clinical Guide to Nutrition Care in Kidney Disease* (pp. 157-188). Academy of Nutrition and Dietetics.

Sethna, C.B., & Gipson, D.S. (2014). Treatment of FSGS in children. *Advances In Chronic Kidney Disease, 21*(2), 194-199. doi:10.1053/j.ackd.2014.01.010

Sutherland, S.M., Zappitelli, M., Alexander, S.R., Chua, A.N., Brophy, P.D., Bunchman, T.E., … Goldstein, S.L. (2010). Fluid overload and mortality in children receiving continuous renal replacement therapy: The prospective pediatric continuous renal replacement therapy registry. *American Journal of Kidney Diseases, 55*(2), 316-325. doi:10.1053/j.ajkd.2009.10.048

Symons, J.M., Chua, A.N., Somers, M.J., Baum, M.A., Bunchman, T.E., Benfield, M.R., … Goldstein, S.L (2007). Demographic characteristics of pediatric continuous renal replacement therapy: A report of the prospective pediatric continuous renal replacement therapy registry. *Clinical Journal of the American Society of Nephrology, 2*(4), 732-738. doi:10.2215/CJN.03200906

Thompson, K.L., Flynn, J.T., Okamura, D., & Zhou, L. (2013). Pretreatment of formula or expressed breast milk with sodium polystyrene sulfonate (Kayexalate) as a treatment for hyperkalemia in infants with acute or chronic renal insufficiency. *Journal of Renal Nutrition, 23*(5), 333-339.

United Network for Organ Sharing (UNOS) (n.d.). *Glossary.* Retrieved from http://optn.transplant.hrsa.gov/resources/glossary.asp

U.S. Renal Data System (USRDS). (2013). *Annual data report: Atlas of chronic kidney disease and end-stage renal disease in the United States.* Bethesda, MD: National Institutes of Health, National Institute of Diabetes and Digestive and Kidney Diseases. Retrieved from http://www.usrds.org/atlas13.aspx

U.S. Renal Data System, (USRDS). (2014). *Annual data report: Atlas of end-stage renal disease in the United States.* Bethesda, MD: National Institutes of Health, National Institute of Diabetes and Digestive and Kidney Diseases. Retrieved from http://www.usrds.org/adr.aspx

Vivante, A., Twig, G., Tirosh, A., Skorecki, K., & Calderon-Margalit, R. (2014). Childhood history of resolved glomerular disease and risk of hypertension during adulthood. *Journal of the American Medical Association, 311*(11):1155-1157. doi:10.1001/jama.2013.284310

Warady, B., Fine, R., Schaefer, F., & Alexander, S. (Eds.). (2004). Pediatric dialysis. Boston: Kluwer Academic Publishers.

Warady, B., Bakkaloglu, S., Newland, J., Cantwell, M., Verrina, E., Neu, A., … Schaefer, F. (2012). ISPD Guidelines/recommendations: Consensus guidelines for the prevention and treatment of catheter-related infections and peritonitis in pediatric patients receiving peritoneal dialysis: 2012 update. *Peritoneal Dialysis International, 32,* S32-S86; doi:10.3747/pdi.2011.00091

Wesseling-Perry, K. (2013). Bone disease in pediatric chronic kidney disease. *Pediatric Nephrology, 28*(4), 569-576.

West, J.B. (2011). *Respiratory physiology – The essentials* (9th ed.). Lippincott Williams & Wilkins.

World Health Organization (WHO). (2010). Annex H, Sexual maturity rating (Tanner Staging) in adolescents. *Antiretroviral therapy for HIV infection in infants and children: Towards universal access: Recommendations for a public health approach: 2010 revision.* Geneva: Author. Retrieved from http://www.ncbi.nlm.nih.gov/books/NBK138588

Care of the Older Adult with Kidney Disease

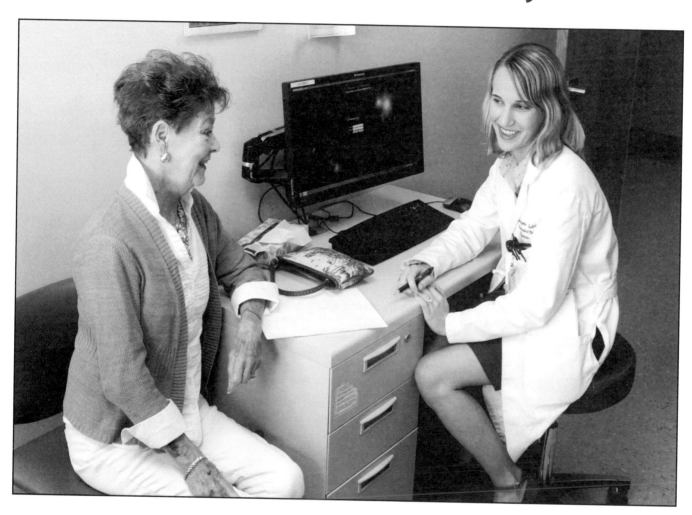

Chapter Editor and Author
Rowena Elliott, PhD, RN, CNN, CNE, AGNP-C, FAAN

CHAPTER **2**
Care of the Older Adult with Kidney Disease

This offering for **1.4 contact hours with 1.0 contact hour of pharmacology content** is provided by the American Nephrology Nurses' Association (ANNA).

American Nephrology Nurses' Association is accredited as a provider of continuing nursing education by the American Nurses Credentialing Center Commission on Accreditation.

ANNA is a provider approved by the California Board of Registered Nursing, provider number CEP 00910.

This CNE offering meets the continuing nursing education requirements for certification and recertification by the Nephrology Nursing Certification Commission (NNCC).

To be awarded contact hours for this activity, read this chapter in its entirety. Then complete the CNE evaluation found at **www.annanurse.org/corecne** and submit it; or print it, complete it, and mail it in. Contact hours are not awarded until the evaluation for the activity is complete.

Example of reference for Chapter 2 in APA format. One author for entire chapter.

Elliott, R. (2015). Care of the older adult with kidney disease. In C.S. Counts (Ed.), *Core curriculum for nephrology nursing: Module 5. Kidney disease in patient populations across the life span* (6th ed., pp. 67-88). Pitman, NJ: American Nephrology Nurses' Association.

Interpreted: Chapter author. (Date). Title of chapter. In …

Cover photo by Counts/Morganello.

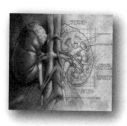

CHAPTER 2

Care of the Older Adult with Kidney Disease

Purpose

The purpose of this chapter is to provide information related specifically to the older adult and kidney disease.

Objectives

Upon completion of this chapter, the learner will be able to:
1. Compare the differences in the leading causes of death in the older adult population between 1900 and 2010.
2. List three physiologic changes that can occur in the older adult.
3. Explain the pharmacokinetic and pharmacodynamic changes that occur in the older adult.
4. Examine the incidence and prevalence of acute kidney injury in the older adult population.
5. Analyze the incidence and prevalence of chronic kidney disease in the older adult population.
6. Explain the benefits and challenges associated with an older adult's choice to receive hemodialysis vs. peritoneal dialysis.

Introduction

With each decade, there has been a steady increase in this population with chronic kidney disease. This chapter provides information related specifically to the older adult and kidney disease. Demographics, physiologic changes, and pharmacologic implications will be discussed. In addition, life expectancy, health promotion, the economic impact of CKD and comorbidities, and the unique challenges associated with addressing issues related to this population and kidney dysfunction will also be presented.

SECTION A
Review of the Aging Process

I. Older adult demographics.

A. In 1900, older adults (65 years of age and older) made up 4.1% of the total population. The percentage rose to 12.4% and 13.0% for 2000 and 2010, respectively. With each decade, there has been a steady increase with the numbers rising to 40.3 million by 2010 (United States Census Bureau, 2011).

B. This represents a 15.1% increase from 2010 when the population was 34.9 million and reflects the largest increase in any decade (see Table 2.1).

C. In 2000, there was a total of 34.9 million people 65 years of age and older. Males made up 41.2% (14,409,625), and the percentage of females was 58.8% (20,582,128).

D. In 2010, there was an increase in the numbers of males and females compared to 2000. The percentage of males was 43.1% (17,362,960) and females were 56.9% (22,905,024).

E. The largest increase was seen in the older adults who were in the age range of 90–94 (see Table 2.2). There was a 30.2% increase for both, 50.3% increase for males, and 23.3% increase for females in the age range. The smallest change occurred with those older adults in the 75–79 age range. There was a decrease in both sexes by 1.3%, an increase for males by 4.5%, and a decrease for females by 5.4% (see Table 2.3).

Table 2.1

United States Population: 65 Years of Age and Older

Year	65 years of age (millions)	Percentage of U. S. population
1900	3.1	4.1
1935	7.8	6.1
1940	9.0	6.8
1950	12.7	8.1
1960	17.2	9.2
1970	20.9	9.9
1980	26.1	11.3
1990	31.9	12.6
2000	34.9	12.4
2010	40.3	13.0

Adapted from "The Older Population: 2010," by the United States Census Bureau, http://www.census.gov/prod/cen2010/briefs/c2010br-09.pdf. Copyright 2011 by the United States Census Bureau.

Table 2.3

Comparison of Male and Female Population: Percent Change from 2000 to 2010

Age	Both Sexes	Male	Female
65–69	30.4	33.0	28.2
70–74	4.7	8.7	1.6
75–79	–1.3	4.5	–5.4
80–84	16.1	25.0	10.9
85–89	29.8	45.3	22.6
90–94'	30.2	50.3	23.3
95–99	5.8	-8.9	9.4

Adapted from "The Older Population: 2010," by the United States Census Bureau, http://www.census.gov/prod/cen2010/briefs/c2010br-09.pdf. Copyright 2011 by the United States Census Bureau.

Table 2.2

Comparison of Male and Female Population (2000 and 2010)

Age	2000			2010		
	Both Sexes	Male	Female	Both Sexes	Male	Female
65-69	9,533,545	4,400,362	5,133,183	12,435,263	5,852,547	6,582,716
70-74	8,857,441	3,902,912	4,954,529	9,278,166	4,243,972	5,034,194
75-79	7,415,813	3,044,456	4,371,357	7,317,795	3,182,388	4,135,407
80-84	4,945,367	1,834,897	3,110,470	5,743,327	2,294,374	3,448,953
85-89	2,789,818	876,501	1,913,317	3,620,459	1,273,867	2,346,592
90-94	1,112,531	282,325	830,206	1,448,366	424,387	1,023,979
95-99	286,784	58,115	228,669	371,244	82,263	288,981
100+	50,454	10,057	40,397	53,364	9,162	44,202
Total	34,991,753 (100%)	14,409,625 (41.2%)	20,582,128 (58.8%)	40,267,984 (100%)	17,362,960 (43.1%)	22,905,024 (56.9%)

Adapted from "The Older Population: 2010," by the United States Census Bureau, http://www.census.gov/prod/cen2010/briefs/c2010br-09.pdf. Copyright 2011 by the United States Census Bureau.

Table 2.4

United States Population: 65 Years of Age and Older by Race

	2009						
Age	**All Races**	**White**	**Black or African American**	**American Indian, Alaska Native**	**Asian**	**Native Hawaiian**	**Hispanic**
65-69	11,784,000	10,068,000	1,092,000	82,000	437,000	13,000	891,000
70-74	9,008,000	7,699,000	843,000	58,000	332,000	10,000	676,000
75-79	7,326,000	6,339,000	644,000	41,000	246,000	7,000	509,000
80-84	5,822,000	5,133,000	451,000	27,000	172,000	4,000	362,000
85-89	3,662,000	3,277,000	247,000	15,000	100,000	2,000	207,000
90-94	1,502,000	1,357,000	89,000	6,000	40,000	1,000	82,000
95-99	402,000	363,000	22,000	2,000	12,000	-----	3,000
100+	64,000	57,000	3,000	-----	3,000	-----	7,000
Total	39,570,000 100%	34,293,000 86.7%	3,391,000 8.57%	231,000 0.58%	1,342,000 3.39%	37,000 0.09%	2.737,000 6.92%

Adapted from "The Older Population: 2010," by the United States Census Bureau, http://www.census.gov/prod/cen2010/briefs/c2010br-09.pdf. Copyright 2011 by the United States Census Bureau.

F. Concerning racial diversity within the population of people 65 years of age and older, a total of 39.5 million older adults represented White, Black (African Americans), Hispanic, American Indians/Alaska Natives, Asian, and Native Hawaiians. White represented 86.7% of the total older adult population. African Americans were 8.57%, followed by Hispanics at 6.92%, and Asians at 3.39% (see Table 2.4).

G. It is projected that 1 in 5 Americans will be 65 years of age or older by 2030 (U.S. Census Bureau, 2010). This progressive increase will have profound implications for all aspects of society, including social, economic, political, and healthcare.

II. Life expectancy.

A. Even though the number of individuals in a specific age-related population increase has a direct effect on society, life expectancy also plays a major role in the rise in the number of individuals 65 years of age and older. The number of years that a group of people will live can assist in planning for healthcare costs.
  1. Life expectancy (at birth) in 1900 was 46.3 years of age for men and 48.3 for women (Centers for Disease Control and Prevention (CDC), 2011).
  2. In 2009, the life expectancy was 76.0 for men and 80.9 for women, an increase of 30.3 and 32.6 years respectively (see Table 2.5).

B. Based on data from the United States Department of Health and Human Services (U. S. DHHS, 2011), there has been a steady increase in life expectancy from 1900 to 2009.
  1. Females have longer life expectancies when compared to men, but the margin has narrowed with each decade.
  2. When comparing life expectancy (at birth), the gap between males and females rose from 2.0 years in 1900 to 7.6 years in 1970.
  3. In contrast, the gap started to narrow after 1970 and dropped to 7.4 years in 1980 and 4.9 years in 2009 (see Table 2.5).

C. When comparing remaining life expectancy (at 65 years of age), the gap between males and females rose from 2.2 years in 1950 to 4.2 years in 1980. The gap narrowed after 1980 and dropped to 2.8 years in 1990 and 2.7 years in 2009.
  1. When adults became 75 years of age, the margins were consistently below 3.0 years. In 1980, a 75-year-old male was expected to live an additional 8.8 years compared to a 75-year-old female who was expected to live an additional 11.5 years – a difference of 2.7 years.

2. By 2009, the gap narrowed to 1.9 years with the life expectancy for males at 86.0 years of age and females at 87.9 years (U. S. DHHS, 2011).

III. Life expectancy: Past, present, and future.

A. In 1900, the life expectancy was an average 47.3 years (male and female), and most adults did not live to the age of 50. During this time, the top three causes of death were pneumonia/influenza, tuberculosis, and gastrointestinal infections (Jones et al., 2012).

1. Immunizations for influenza and pneumonia, antibiotics, and tuberculosis screenings were not in existence in 1900.

2. Penicillin, the first antibiotic, was discovered in 1928 and developed for medical use in 1940 (CDC, 1999).

3. The influenza vaccine was not available until 1945 (National Network for Immunization Information, 2010a), and the pneumococcal vaccine was not licensed until 1977 (National Network for Immunization Information, 2010b).

4. The Mantoux tuberculosis screening test was first created in 1907, and the first successful treatment for tuberculosis, streptomycin, wasn't administered until 1944 (New Jersey Medical School Global Tuberculosis Institute, 2012).

5. Without this protection and treatment modalities, the death rates were substantially higher and people succumbed to these conditions which are currently preventable and treatable. For example, in 1918, the influenza flu pandemic resulted in a 10-year decrease in life expectancy (CDC, 2012). After the influenza immunization became available in 1945, the life expectancy started to rise.

B. In 2010, 110 years later, the top three causes of death were heart disease, cancer, and chronic pulmonary diseases (CDC, 2012) (see Table 2.6).

1. The primary causes of death in 1900

Table 2.5

Remaining Life Expectancy

Year	At birth	At 65 years of age	At 75 years of age
1900	Male – 46.3 Female – 48.3	N/A*	N/A*
1950	Male – 65.6 Female – 71.7	Male (Male (+12.8) = 77.8 Female (+15.0) = 80.0	
1960	Male – 66.6 Female – 73.1	Male (Male (+12.8) = 77.8 Female (+15.8) = 80.8	
1970	Male – 67.1 Female – 74.7	Male (Male (+13.1) = 78.1 Female (+17.0) = 82.0	
1980	Male – 70.0 Female – 77.4	Male (Male (+14.1) = 79.1 Female (+18.3) = 83.3	Male (+8.8) = 83.8 Female (+11.5) = 86.5
1990	Male – 71.8 Female – 78.8	Male (Male (+15.1) = 80.1 Female (+18.9) = 83.9	Male (+9.4) = 84.4 Female (+12.0) = 87.0
2000	Male – 74.1 Female – 79.3	Male (Male (+16.0) = 81.0 Female (+19.0) = 84.0	Male (+9.8) = 84.8 Female (+11.8) = 86.8
2009	Male – 76.0 Female – 80.9	Male (Male (+17.6) = 82.6 Female (+20.3) = 85.3	Male (+11.0) = 86.0 Female (+12.9) = 87.9

Adapted from "Life Expectancy," by the Centers for Disease Control and Prevention, http://www.cdc.gov/nchs/fastats/lifexpec.htm. Copyright 2011 by the Centers for Disease Control and Prevention.

Table 2.6

10 Leading Causes of Death for Persons 65 years of Age and Older for 2010 and 2012

1	Heart disease	Heart disease
2	Cancer	Cancer
3	Noninfectious airway diseases	Chronic lower respiratory disease
4	Cerebrovascular disease	Cerebrovascular disease
5	Accidents	Alzheimer's disease
6	Alzheimer's disease	Diabetes mellitus
7	Diabetes mellitus	Influenza and pneumonia
8	Nephropathies	Nephritis, nephrotic syndrome, nephrosis
9	Pneumonia or influenza	Accidents
10	Suicide	Septicemia

Adapted from "Deaths and Mortality," by the Centers for Disease Control and Prevention, http://www.cdc.gov/nchs/fastats/death.htm. Copyright 2010 by the Centers for Disease Control and Prevention. Also used as source: "The Burden of Disease and the Changing Task of Medicine," by D. S. Jones & J. A. Green, 2012, *New England Journal of Medicine, 366*, pp. 2333-2338. Copyright 2012 by the *New England Journal of Medicine*.

were directly related to an infectious process that did not have a treatment or cure.

2. In contrast, two of the primary causes of death in 2010, heart disease and chronic obstructive pulmonary disease, can be directly related to lifestyle choices.

3. With the increase in the dietary consumption of foods that raise cholesterol levels (e.g., LDL, triglycerides) and blood pressure levels, more sedentary lifestyles, and the glamorization of cigarette and cigar smoking, there has been a rise in the incidence and prevalence of medical conditions related to these modern lifestyles.

C. A study by Danaei et al. (2010) found there is a direct correlation between exposure to four preventable risk factors (smoking, hypertension, hyperglycemia, and obesity), individual and community characteristics, and reduced life expectancy in 2005.

1. For example, Western Native Americans and low income African Americans in the rural south had the highest probability of dying between 15 and 60 years of age due to cardiovascular disease and cancer. However, White and Native American women had higher rates of mortality directly related to smoking.

2. The researchers suggested that reduction in these risk factors could increase the probability of adding more years to life expectancy. The authors added that implementation of health promotion and prevention policies and programs should be directed at specific vulnerable populations.

3. Although the basic healthy habits are listed as (a) no smoking, (b) 30 minutes of moderate exercise five times a week, (c) consuming five servings of fruits and vegetables daily, and (d) maintaining a normal body weight, only 3% of the U.S.

population follow the recommended guidelines (Desai et al., 2010; EDTNA, 2011).

4. According to Curry (2008), approximately 90% of older adults never receive routine screening tests for bone density, colon cancer, or glaucoma. In addition, approximately 60% do not receive preventive screening for hypertension and hyperlipidemia (see Table 2.7).

Table 2.7

Immunization and Screening Guidelines for Older Adults (including those with chronic illness)

Immunization /Screening	Guidelines
Influenza	Annually at the beginning of flu season (November).
Pneumovax	Once after 65 years old; Booster after 5 years if initial was before 65 years old.
Tetanus, diptheria, pertussis	Booster every 10 years. Adults 50 years or older should receive one dose of Td regardless of time since last immunization.
Zoster	Indicated for adults 60 years or older (regardless if they report a prior episode of shingles). Must have a history of chickenpox or varicella before giving the vaccine.
Hepatitis A and B	Recommended only if risk factors are present.
Measles, mumps, rubella	Recommended only if risk factors are present.
Varicella	If there is lack of immunity and risk for exposure.
Fecal occult blood and rectal exam	Annually.
Sigmoidoscopy or colonoscopy	Every 5–10 years at 50–75 years of age.
Diabetes mellitus	Every 3 years. More frequently if risk factors are present.
Eye exam	Annual acuity and glaucoma screening.
Tobacco	Provide interventions for smoking cessation.
Depression	Annually with Geriatric Depression Scale.
Dental exams/screenings	Annually for those with teeth, cleaning every 6 months, and every 2 years for denture wearers.
Prostate surface antigen (PSA)	> 50 years old or 45 years old if risk factors are present.
Mammogram	Every 1–2 years if > 40 years old.
Pap smear and pelvic examination	Every 3 years. Can stop pap smears at age 65 if three negative tests in the past 10 years.

Adapted from "Disease Prevention and Health Promotion for Older Adults," by T. A. Touhy & K. Jett, 2012, Ebersole & Hess' Toward Healthy Aging: Human Needs & Nursing Response. Copyright 2012 by Elsevier Mosby.

IV. Physiologic changes in the older adult. As the body increases in age, various age-related changes can occur.

A. These changes occur to varying degrees, depending on the older adult's past lifestyle habits, medical history, genetics, and environment.

B. Appendix 2.1 lists and describes the age-related changes that occur in various physiologic systems of the body.

V. Pharmacologic changes in the older adult.

A. With the increasing population of older adults, subsequent increase in the incidence and prevalence of chronic illness, and increase in the number and types of drugs used (prescribed, over-the-counter, and herbal supplements), there is also the need for nurses to be aware of the pharmacologic changes that occur in the older adult population.
1. Adults older than 65 years of age make up about 13% of the population. However, this population consumes over 33% of all prescription medications and 40% of all over-the-counter (OTC) medications (Adams et al., 2013).
2. More than 40% of men and women over the age of 65 take five or more medications weekly, and 12% take 10 or more medications weekly (Tablowski, 2014). According to Planton and Edlund (2010), the use of multiple medications or using multiple medications simultaneously is defined as polypharmacy.
3. Polypharmacy can increase the risk for morbidity and mortality in the older adult when combined with multiple medical conditions, lower physiologic reserves, decreased kidney and liver function, and cognitive impairment (Mauk, 2014).
4. These statistics regarding medication use in the older adult can present various challenges that include normal age-related changes, chronic medical conditions, cognitive changes, psychosocial variables, and acute medical issues that may arise at any time.
5. In addition to addressing these interrelated challenges, the nurse must have knowledge of the numerous pharmacokinetics and pharmacodynamics changes that can occur as one ages. This is necessary when prescribing, administering, and monitoring medications.

B. Pharmacokinetics refers to what the human body does to a drug. It includes absorption, distribution, metabolism, and excretion, all of which are affected by the aging process. See Table 2.8 for a list of pharmacokinetics in the older adult, physiologic effects, and possible drug responses.

Table 2.8

Pharmacokinetics in the Older Adult

Phases	Physiologic Effects and Possible Drug Responses
Absorption	Decrease in gastric acidity (increased pH) alters absorption of weak acids such as aspirin.
	Increased alkaline gastric secretions allows for enteric-coated drugs to dissolve more rapidly.
	Decrease in blood flow to the GI tract (40–50% less) is caused by a decrease in cardiac output. Because of reduced blood flow, absorption is slowed, but not decreased.
	Reduction in peristalsis may delay onset of action.
	Reduction in gastric emptying occurs.
Distribution	Because of a decrease in body water, water-soluble drugs are more concentrated.
	Increase in fat-to-water ratio in older adult. Fat soluble drugs are stored and likely to accumulate (example: diazepam/Valium®).
	Decrease in circulating serum protein (esp. albumin and alpha-1 acid glycoprotein). Acidic drugs (NSAIDs, aspirin, benzodiazepines, phenytoin, and warfarin) bind to albumin. Beta blockers, tricyclic antidepressants and lidocaine bind to alpha-1 acid glycoprotein.
	With fewer protein-binding sites, there is more free drug available to body tissue at receptor sites.
	Drugs with a high affinity for protein (> 90%) compete for protein binding sites with other drugs.
	Drug interactions and toxicity result because of lack of protein sites and increase in free drugs.
Metabolism	Decrease in hepatic enzyme production, hepatic blood flow (40%–45%), liver size, and total liver function. These decreases cause a reduction in drug metabolism.
	With reduction in metabolic rate, the half-life of drugs increase, and drug accumulation can result.
	Metabolism of drug inactivates drug/drug metabolite and prepares it for elimination via the kidneys.
	When drug clearance by the liver is decreased, half life is longer, when drug clearance is increased, half-life is shortened. With prolonged half-life, accumulation can result and drug toxicity could occur.
Excretion	Decrease in renal blood flow and decrease in GFR or 40-50%. With decrease in kidney function comes decrease in drug excretion and drug accumulation results.
	Drug toxicity should be assessed continually while the older adult takes the drug.

1. Absorption – movement of a drug from the site of administration, across biologic barriers, and into the plasma.
2. Distribution – movement of a drug from the plasma into the cells.
3. Metabolism – when drugs are transformed into an inactive state.
4. Excretion – release of drug metabolites from the body.

C. Pharmacodynamics refers to what the drug does to the body. This includes the intended action, side effects, adverse effects, and allergic reactions.
1. Intended actions – desired effect that improves body function.
2. Side effect – one or more effects on body cells or tissues that are not the intended action.
3. Adverse effect – harmful side effect that is more severe than expected and has potential to damage tissue or cause serious health problems.
4. Allergic reaction – type of adverse effect in which the presence of the drug stimulates the release of histamine and other substances that cause inflammatory reactions.

D. It is important to note that caution should be exercised when prescribing, administering, and monitoring drugs to minimize side effects and avoid adverse effects.
1. There is minimal evidence in the research to validate some of the issues that can occur with older adults and drugs.
2. A variety of drugs that were approved by the U.S. Food and Drug Administration (FDA) before 1989 were not studied in the older adult population (Tablowski, 2014).
3. Since 1989, the FDA has required that drugs be studied in the older adult population and the results included in the Geriatric Considerations section of drug inserts.

E. Although advances have been made to include older adults in drug studies, there is still concern that those older than 85 years of age are not included in drug studies.
1. Efforts to include all ages in drug studies are progressing.
2. However, the nurse also should be aware that chronologic age alone does not predict the specific pharmacokinetics and pharmacodynamics on an older adult.
3. Other variables that are just as vital in predicting drug action.
   a. The older adult's state of health.
   b. The number and types of other medications taken.
   c. Kidney and liver function.

(1) As the liver ages, there is a decrease in the size of the liver, blood flow to the organ, and number of enzymes. As a result, there is a decrease and delay in drug metabolism. These age-related changes can increase the risk for drug toxicities (Tablowski, 2014).
(2) As the kidney ages, there is a decrease in the size of the kidneys, blood flow to the organs, and glomerular filtration rate. These age-related changes can lead to elevated serum drug levels and toxicities (Tablowski, 2014.)
   d. The presence of other medical conditions.
   e. Comorbidities or chronic conditions.

VI. Chronic illness in the older adult.

A. Chronic illness, chronic medical conditions, and chronic health problems are terms used to describe health problems that have slow, progressive, and insidious onsets.
1. The above-mentioned conditions are usually identified:
   a. Through a health screening. For example, an older adult may attend a health screening, and elevated BUN and creatinine levels may be identified leading to a diagnosis of chronic kidney disease stage 3.
   b. While a person is being treated for another medical issue. For example, an older adult may have a diagnosis of hypertension. During the course of treatment, chronic kidney disease (a chronic illness) is diagnosed due to the long-term effects of hypertension on the kidney tissue. These long-term effects include inflammation and ischemia, which cause a decrease in filtration (McCance & Huether, 2010; Touhy & Jett, 2012).
2. It is important to note that the presence of a chronic illness is not as important as its effect on function and ability to carry out activities of daily living (ADLs) and instrumental activities of daily living (IADLs).
3. Some older adults with chronic conditions may be able to continue their present lifestyle. However, with advancing age, the effects may restrict functional status (Touhy & Jett, 2012).

B. In 2007 and 2008, the leading chronic illnesses among the population of men and women who are 65 years of age and older were hypertension, arthritis, heart disease, cancer (any type), diabetes, asthma, chronic bronchitis or emphysema, and stroke. Hypertension was the most common.
1. Older women had a greater rate of hypertension, arthritis, asthma, and chronic bronchitis/emphysema.

2. Men had higher rates of heart disease, cancer (any type), and diabetes.

3. The rates of stroke were the same between men and women (Touhy & Jett, 2012).

4. Just 4 years later in 2012, the list changed to include visual, hearing, and orthopedic impairments (Eliopoulos, 2014).

C. The majority of older adults have at least one chronic illness, but more often they have more than one chronic illness, known as comorbidities.

1. When an individual has comorbidities, simultaneous management of care for several chronic conditions is needed.

2. The nurse who is providing care for the older adult with a chronic illness has an opportunity to help decrease the mortality and minimize the disabling effects of chronic disease while helping to decrease morbidity (Touhy & Jett, 2012).

3. One of the challenges of the nurse is to develop and implement strategies that will promote healthy aging in the presence of chronic diseases like chronic kidney disease.

D. In an effort to assist healthcare professionals to understand the realities of chronic illness and its effect on individuals, Corbin and Strauss (1992) conceptualized a trajectory model for chronic illnesses (see Table 2.9).

Table 2.9

Stages of Chronic Illness Trajectory

Pre-trajectory	Before the illness course begins, the preventive phase, no signs or symptoms are present.
Trajectory onset	Signs and symptoms are present, includes diagnostic period.
Crisis	Life threatening situation, acute threat to self-identity.
Acute	Active illness or complications that require hospitalization for management.
Stable	Controlled illness course/symptoms.
Unstable	Illness course/symptoms not controlled by regimen but not requiring or desiring hospitalization
Downward	Progressive decline in physical/mental status characterized by increasing disability/symptoms
Dying	Immediate weeks, days, hours preceding death.

1. According to the Chronic Illness Trajectory, chronic illness can be viewed from a life course perspective or along a trajectory. By using this view, the course of a person's illness can be seen as an integral part of their lives instead of an isolated event. Hence, the nurse's response will be holistic rather that episodic and isolated (Touhy & Jett, 2012).

2. This trajectory is divided into eight phases with the intent to identify goals and develop interventions that are individualized for the individual and his/her significant others. Key points of the model are based on theoretical assumptions and are listed below (Woog, 1992).

a. The majority of health problems in late life are chronic.

b. Chronic illnesses may entail lifetime adaptations.

c. Chronic illnesses and their management often profoundly affect the lives and identities of both the individual and the family members or significant others.

d. The acute phase of management is designed to stabilize physiologic processes and promote recovery.

E. Other phases of management are designed primarily to maximize and extend the period of stability in the home with the help of family and by visits to and from healthcare providers and other members of the rehabilitation and restoration team as appropriate.

F. A primary care nurse is often in the role of coordinator of the multiple resources that may be needed to promote quality of life along the trajectory.

G. The nurse has multiple resources that may be needed to promote quality of life along the trajectory.

H. The nurse has multiple opportunities to promote the health of persons during the chronic phase.

Section B
Kidney Disease in the Older Adult

I. Kidney disease and the older adult.

A. There is an age-related decline in kidney function which results in impaired ability to concentrate urine, conserve sodium and water, adjust to rapid hemodynamic changes, and maintain homeostasis with fluid and electrolyte levels. Approximately 30% of individuals who are over the age of 70 and 50%

Table 2.10

Kidney Diagnostic Parameters in the Older Adult

Diagnostic Test	Rationale	Adult	Older Adult	Implications
Kidney Ultrasound	Kidney weight decrease 20–40% between the ages of 30 and 90	Kidney length – 9 cm Abnormal – Less than 9 cm or a difference of 1.5 cm	Decrease in kidney length by 2 cm	Decrease in size of kidneys in the older adult does not necessarily imply chronicity as it would in the adult.
Serum Creatinine	Decreased muscle mass and diminished production of endogenous creatinine	Age 40–60 Male 1.1–1.5 mg/dL Female 1.0–0.97 mg.dL	Age 60-99 Male 1.5-1.20 mg/dL Female 0.99-0.91 mg/dL	Serum creatinine cannot be used as a marker for kidney function in the older adult.
Creatinine Clearance	Age-related reduction in kidney plasma flow and glomerular filtration rate	140 mL/min/1,73 m²	97 mL/min/1.73 m²	Cockcroft and Gault formula should be used to determine Cr clearance (kidney function) in the older adult.
Urine Osmolarity	Tubular function decreases, causing less effective concentration of urine	1,109 mOsm/kg	882 mOsm/kg	Measurement of urine osmolality is of limited value in differentiating prerenal azotemia and acute tubular necrosis in the older adult.
Fractional excretion of sodium (FENa+)	Decreased capacity to reabsorb sodium by the ascending loop of Henle	Prerenal < 1% Intrinsic > 1%	Not reliable values	Cannot be used to differentiate azotemia and acute tubular necrosis in the older adult.
Glomerular filtration rate (GFR)	Decreased kidney mass and filtration rate	90–140 mL/min	< 75 mL/min by the age of 70	Same parameters are used to diagnose stages of CKD, although an age-related decrease may not be considered when diagnosing.

Adapted from Counts., C.S. (2008). *Core curriculum for nephrology nursing* (5th ed.) Pitman, NJ: American Nephrology Nurses' Association.

over age 80 have abnormal kidney function (Weiss et al., 2011).

B. If abnormal signs and symptoms are present, they are usually atypical for kidney disease and are frequently attributed to pre-existing conditions. Hence, kidney disease may go undetected and undiagnosed in the older adult.
   1. Serum creatinine may remain in the normal range despite the age-related decline in GFR due to age-related loss of muscle mass and decrease in protein intake.
   2. A creatinine clearance is the most accurate test for assessment of kidney function, but if the levels are low, it should be evaluated and not dismissed as an age-related value (Samiy, 1983).
   3. Additional age-related changes to the kidney and

other systems can affect diagnostic parameters (see Table 2.10).

II. Acute renal failure/acute kidney injury: Incidence and prevalence.

A. The rate of acute kidney injury (AKI) in Medicare patients who were 66 to 69 years of age in 2011 was 14.9 per 1000 patient years (United States Renal Data Set (USRDS), 2012).

B. The rates were higher for those 70 to 74 years of age (18.8); 75 to 79 years of age (26.4); 80 to 84 years of age (35.9); and 85+ years of age (49.6).

C. The incidence of Medicare patients 66 years of age and older also varied according to race in 2011.

D. Blacks/African Americans had a rate of 45.3 per 1000 patient hours followed by Whites (25.8) and other races (23.9).

E. Based on these statistics, Blacks/African Americans and those 85+ years of age had the highest incidence of AKI (see Table 2.11).

III. Chronic kidney disease: Incidence and prevalence.

A. Heart disease, cardiovascular disease, and diabetes mellitus are the primary risk factors for development of chronic kidney disease (USRDS, 2012) and are in the top 10 causes of death in the United States (refer to Table 2.6).

B. The United States Renal Data Set (USRDS) developed the 2012 annual report describing various aspects of chronic kidney disease.
   1. This survey data was obtained in 2010 using the National Health and Nutrition Survey (NHANES) and used a random population of approximately 27 million participants.
   2. According to the National Kidney Foundation (2012), CKD is defined as an estimated glomerular filtration rate (GFR) less than 60 mL/min/1.73 m^2 or urine albumin to creatinine ratio (ACR) of > 30 mg/G or higher. This data is used to determine the five stages of CKD (USRDS, 2012).

C. The data for the year 2010 showed that 1.2 million of the participants were identified as 65 years of age or older and receiving Medicare benefits with a mean age of 75.3. Within this population, there were 112,308 individuals with a diagnosis of CKD (stages 1 to 5); the mean age was 77.9.
   1. For the older adults (65+) with CKD, 36.9% were 65 to 74 years old; 41.2% were 75 to 84 years of age; and 21.9% were 85 years and older (see Table 2.12).
   2. When considering risk factors that contribute to CKD, this population of older adults had a diagnosis of CKD in addition to diabetes mellitus (47.6%), hypertension (92.2%), and congestive heart failure (31.8%).
   3. It is also noted that this data reflects a threefold increase in older adults diagnosed with CKD from 2000–2010 (USRDS, 2012).
   4. According to the USRDS (2014), the prevalence of CKD in those individuals 60 years of age and older was 32.2% (1988–1994), 37.5 % (1999–2004), and 33.2% (2007–2012).

D. This steady increase in the older adult population and increase in those older adults diagnosed with

---

Table 2.11

Unadjusted Rates of First AKI within the Cohort Year (2011) among Medicare Patients Age 66 and Older (per 1000 patient years)

Year	White	Black/African-American	Other Races
1996	2.9	6.2	3.1
2001	5.7	11.9	6.9
2006	13.0	26.6	13.2
2011	25.8	45.3	23.9

Table 2.12

Older Adults and Chronic Kidney Disease (CKD)

Age	CKD Population (thousands)	Percentage of CKD Population (65+)
65-74	41,442	36.9
75-84	46,271	41.2
85+	24,595	21.9

Adapted from "2012 Annual Data Report: Atlas of Chronic Kidney Disease and End-Stage Renal Disease in the United States," by the United States Renal Data System, http://www.usrds.org/adr.aspx. Copyright 2011 by United States Renal Data System.

CKD presents a concern and challenge when promoting health promotion and disease prevention. This is especially true when faced with the related costs to the Medicare program and the effect it has on the current and future economy.

E. Medicare is a federally funded insurance program for individuals 65 years of age and older, those under 65 with qualifying disabilities, and any age with a diagnosis of end stage renal disease (ESRD) (Centers for Medicare and Medicaid [CMS], 2012).
   1. There are criteria to be eligible for Medicare. They include:
      a. A United States citizen or permanent legal resident.
      b. The individual or spouse has earned 40 credits (approximately 10 years of employment) and is eligible for Social Security or railroad retirement benefits.
      c. Individual or spouse has paid Medicare payroll taxes while working.

2. Medicare's total expenditures are approximately 241 billion dollars annually. According to the USRDS (2012), individuals (65+) with a diagnosis of CKD account for 17% of the total Medicare expenditures (41 billion dollars).
3. Older adults with CKD and diabetes used 22.1 billion of the 42 billion dollars. This is alarming because it represents the impact that one chronic medical condition can have on an entire country's health and economy.

IV. Acute renal failure/acute kidney injury in the older adult.

A. Acute kidney injury occurs when there is a rapid reduction in kidney function that results in a failure to maintain fluid, electrolyte, and acid-base homeostasis (Lewington & Kanagasundaram, 2011).
1. It has replaced the term acute renal failure because it enables healthcare professionals to consider, treat, and monitor the disease as a spectrum of injury instead of a condition that reflects coexisting pathologies.
2. This new paradigm was developed upon finding that small increases in serum creatinine levels are corresponding to poor clinical outcomes (Lewington & Kanagasundaram, 2011).
3. This has initiated collaborative efforts to develop a universal definition of AKI and develop global guidelines to assess, diagnose, and treat acute kidney injury (Lewington & Kanagasundaram, 2011).

B. Acute kidney injury is especially important to the older adult population because these individuals are vulnerable and at an increased risk for developing this condition. According to Lewington & Kanagasundaram (2011), the risk factors for developing acute kidney injury include:
1. Age > 75 years.
2. Chronic kidney disease (eGFR < 60 mL/min/1.73 m²).
3. Heart failure.
4. Atherosclerotic peripheral vascular disease.
5. Liver disease.
6. Diabetes mellitus.
7. Nephrotoxic drugs.

C. In the older adult population, AKI is usually associated with factors which include preexisting renal dysfunction, heart failure, atherosclerotic renal artery stenosis, exposure to radiographic dyes, and use of various nephrotoxic drugs (nonsteroidal antiinflammatory drugs, ACE inhibitors, and diuretics) (Cheung et al., 2008). The etiology is currently categorized as prerenal, intrarenal/intrinsic, and postrenal.

1. Prerenal AKI is the second most common cause in the older adult and accounts for nearly 33% of all hospitalized cases. Prerenal causes include:
   a. True volume depletion (e.g., decreased fluid intake).
   b. Decreased effective blood volume (e.g., systemic vasodilation).
   c. Hemodynamic (e.g., renal artery stenosis).
2. The intrarenal/intrinsic causes include, most commonly, acute tubular necrosis (ATN), which accounts for 50% of hospitalized patients with AKI and 76% of cases in patients in the intensive care unit.
   a. Acute tubular necrosis is the accumulation of myeloid (protein) bodies in the kidney tubules.
   b. ATN can be induced by drugs, such as aminoglycosides.
3. Postrenal causes commonly found in the older adult include:
   a. Benign prostatic hypertrophy.
   b. Prostatic carcinoma.
   c. Pelvic malignancies (Cheung et al., 2008).

D. When considering the risk factors and causes of AKI, it is vital for the interdisciplinary team to obtain a comprehensive medical and drug history in addition to a physical exam. (Refer to Module 4 on acute kidney injury.)

E. For those older adults (66+) who required dialysis, intermittent hemodialysis (IHD) was the most common treatment modality.
1. In 2011, 36% of AKI patients were placed on IHD compared to 65% in 2000. This reflects a decline in the use of IHD as a dialysis modality.
2. Daily hemodialysis was the second most common, and continuous hemodialysis was used least (USRDS, 2012).

F. There is not a great deal of difference in the general principles for treating AKI in the older adult when compared to other populations.
1. However, priority should be placed on addressing life-threatening issues, such as shock, respiratory failure, hyperkalemia, pulmonary edema, metabolic acidosis, and sepsis.
2. Hemodynamic and fluid status should be routinely monitored and nephrotoxins should be discontinued.
3. Pharmacists should be consulted so drug dosages and scheduling can be adjusted to avoid possible toxicities.
4. Nutritional assessment and support should be included in the treatment plan.
5. One of the most important and integral elements of the treatment plan should include early referral to a nephrologist to accurately determine the cause

of AKI and to initiate and individualize treatment in a timely manner (Cheung et al., 2008).

G. Following hospitalization to treat AKI, the probability of a recurrent AKI event within 12 months did not vary greatly with age, regardless whether dialysis was part of the treatment plan (USRDS, 2012, 2014).
 1. According to USRDS (2012) data, there was a change in the CKD stage upon discharge after the initial diagnosis of AKI. For those who were at stage 1–2 prior to hospitalization, 45% were classified as stage 3–5 CKD upon discharge. For those who were classified as stage 3–5 CKD before hospitalization, 11.5% changed to CKD Stage 5 (ESRD) upon discharge.
 2. Similar changes occurred in those who had a recurrent hospitalization after the initial diagnosis of AKI. For those with CKD stages 1-2, 50% were later classified as having stages 3–5 CKD upon discharge.
 3. Of older adults with stages 3–5 CKD, 9.2% were reclassified as stage 5 CKD/ESRD after hospitalization (USRDS, 2012).

H. It is important to note that although comprehensive and intense assessment, diagnosis, and treatment can be performed, mortality from AKI has not changed to a significant degree in the past 40 years. The mortality rate is currently up to 75% (Cheung et al., 2008).

V. Chronic kidney disease (CKD) in the older adult.

A. Approximately 16.5% of the U.S. population (20 years of age and older) are affected by CKD stages 1 to 5 (USRDS, 2012).
 1. This percentage is substantially higher in older adults who are 70 years of age and older (30%) and those 80 years of age and older (50%).
 2. These are alarming statistics that warrant the need for healthcare providers to be competent and skilled to manage all of the various health challenges that are present with a diagnosis of CKD.
 3. Most of the care used for older adults with CKD is actually more applicable to the younger adult and does not consider the age-related physical, environmental, and social issues that are specific to the older individuals. In light of this, an age-specific approach could be a major benefit (Weiss, Petrik, & Thorp, 2011).
 4. It is also important to note that age should not be the sole factor in developing a treatment and management plan. Other important factors include functional status and desired outcomes (American Nurses Association, 2010).

B. Early referral of the older adult to a nephrologist is beneficial.
 1. The evidence shows that early referral to nephrology and management of comorbidities (anemia, malnutrition, and heart disease) could result in improved survival for patients who start kidney replacement therapy.
 2. Current guidelines for primary care providers do not consider the complexities of the older adult with CKD, which include:
  a. Functional loss.
  b. Cognitive impairment.
  c. Additional comorbidities (Bowling & O'Hare, 2012; Campbell et al., 2008).

C. Other factors that have an impact on decision making include the patient's perceptions of the disease, his/her emotional reaction to the diagnosis, adherence to the current treatment regimen, and realistic and unrealistic expectations (Campbell, 2008).

D. Since the complexities of the older adult with CKD (functional loss, cognitive impairment, geriatric syndromes, and additional long-term complications of CKD) play a major role in treatment regimens and outcomes, Bowling & O'Hare (2012) have suggested the use of an individualized patient-centered model of care.
 1. This model of care prioritizes patient preferences and embraces the notion that observed signs and symptoms often do not reflect a single underlying disease process but reflect the complex interplay between many different factors. It emphasizes modifiable outcomes that matter to the patient.
 2. Information related to patient preferences and outcomes are used to shape rather than dictate care. The authors stated that this model of care may have more benefits to the older adult with CKD compared to the traditional disease-oriented approach.

E. The disease-oriented model of care.
 1. Assumes a direct causal association between observed signs and symptoms and underlying disease processes.
 2. Treatment plans using this model target disease processes with the goal of improving disease-related outcomes.

F. It is important to note that the disease-oriented approach has been used extensively and effectively in the renal community with the development, dissemination, and revisions of the practice guidelines. It has also been very useful in establishing a universal definition of CKD.
 1. However, the authors suggest that a different

model be adopted when developing the plan of care for the older adult with CKD.

2. The challenge that occurs when using the disease-oriented model of care for an older adult is directly related to the presence of comorbidities with this population.

3. When older adults have multiple comorbid conditions, some of the treatment guidelines may have similar treatments and outcomes while others may have opposing treatment guidelines.

4. For example, an older adult may have diabetes, vascular disease, and hypertension. The treatment guidelines will be similar for these conditions. However, the same older adult may have osteoarthritis, and the pain medication may be nephrotoxic.

5. These potential conflicts and challenges are the premise for using a patient-centered model of care.

VI. Choice of dialysis modality and the older adult.

A. Factors the patient, family, and healthcare providers should consider when the time comes for the older adult to choose a dialysis modality.
   1. Impact on the individual's lifestyle, social environment, personality, and health status.
   2. Impact the modality will have on the older adult's quality of life and level of independence.
   3. Whether the choice is peritoneal dialysis or hemodialysis, it should be made by a well-informed patient with preferences respected and incorporation of family input, as appropriate (EDTNA, 2011).

B. When considering best outcomes for peritoneal dialysis and hemodialysis, several studies have been conducted to explore which is best for the older adult.
   1. The North Thames Dialysis Study (Lamping, 2000) compared outcomes of older adults (> 70 years of age) who were receiving PD and HD. There was no significant difference in survival and quality of life between PD and HD.
   2. In the BOLDE study (Brown & Johansson, 2010), the results showed that in two groups of older adults on HD and PD, health-related quality of life was similar.
   3. Some of the variables that affect selection of a modality include:
      a. Physician preference (nephrologist and primary care).
      b. Patient and family preference.
      c. Functional status.
      d. Environmental and home status.
      e. Cognitive status.

   f. Social support systems.
   g. Vascular system status.
   h. Cardiac status.
   i. Pulmonary status.
   j. History of surgical procedures (e.g., abdominal) (Counts, 2008).

VII. Special considerations for the older adult receiving peritoneal dialysis.

A. Peritoneal dialysis provides better cardiovascular homeostasis, longer residual kidney function, and fewer complications with fluid volume imbalances for the older adult.
   1. Water and solutes are removed more slowly and there is reduced risk for arrhythmias related to cardiovascular instability.
   2. If the older adult has pre-existing vascular deficiencies, it may not be feasible for the patient to have a fistula of graft for hemodialysis. Therefore, peritoneal dialysis may be the better option.
   3. Advantages of using PD as a dialysis modality for the older adult include more liberal fluid intake, reduced costs, and fewer transportation issues (EDTNA, 2011).
   4. Older age, mental inability, or poor adherence should not be contraindication for PD; however, they should be considered and addressed if this is the modality choice.
   5. Whether age-related or secondary to a medical condition, visual impairment, tremor, and deformities of the hand may interfere with handling PD supplies and equipment.
   6. Actions should be taken to adapt the training so the older adult can maintain as much independence as possible.

B. See Table 2.13 for points to consider when conducting PD training for the older adult.

VIII. Special considerations for the older adult receiving hemodialysis.

A. Although advancing age should not prevent an older adult from receiving a vascular access, it should be noted that this population is more likely to have less than optimum vasculature for use with hemodialysis.
   1. Atheromas and calcifications may further compromise vasculature.
   2. Regardless of age, the arteriovenous fistula (AVF) is the first choice for a vascular access, followed by the arteriovenous graft (AVG).
   3. The central venous catheter should always be the last resort due to increased infection and mortality rates.

Table 2.13

Points to Consider When Conducting Peritoneal Dialysis Training for the Older Adult

Hearing	If the patient wears a hearing aid, make sure it is available and in good working order.
	Speak slowly and distinctly, but do not shout.
	Face the patient because her or she may read lips.
Vision	If the patient wears corrective lenses, make sure they are available and clean.
	Ensure adequate lighting and incorporate as much natural light as possible.
	Consider age-related light sensitivity (glare) and problems with color perceptions (use contrasting colors, if possible).
	Use large print reading materials.
Temperature Control	Older adults are more likely to feel cold. Adjust the temperature for patient comfort.
Learning ability	Information may be processed slowly, so be patient and repeat the information as needed.
	Use different formats to present the information.
	Provide review questions (verbally or written).
	Allow the older adult time to ask questions.
	Use simple terms and try to avoid medical terminology.
	Keep in mind that some older adults have computer skills, but adapt the teaching session if they do not have computer skills.
Cognition	If the older adult has cognitive disorders, make sure teaching periods are provided in short time periods of 10-15 minutes.
Functional Challenges	When deciding on the type of PD to be used, dexterity challenges (arthritis, decreased muscle strength, etc.) must be considered.
Family and Significant Others	Include family and significant others in the teaching session, but ensure that the older adult's independence and decision-making is honored.

Adapted from European Dialysis and Transplantation Nurses Association (2011). *Caring for the elderly renal patient: A guide to clinical practice.* Luzern, Switzerland: EDTNA/ERCA.

B. Quality of life is a very important factor when the older adult is deciding on treatment modality.
  1. More older adults chose hemodialysis for relief of symptoms as opposed to survival.
  2. Factors that may have a negative impact on quality of life for the older adult receiving hemodialysis include:
     a. Intradialytic hypotension related to removal of too much fluid during hemodialysis.
     b. Functional impairment such as arthritis or other physical limitations.
     c. Failure of the vascular access due to age-related changes on the vasculature (e.g., stiff less elastic arteries and vein).
     d. Frequent hospitalizations related to clot formation in the vascular access, infection, or complications from comorbid conditions (American Nephrology Nurses' Association, 2008).

iX. Care considerations.

A. It is imperative for nurses to realize how important it is to become familiar with the care that is needed for this unique population of patients.

B. The next step in acquisition of information and application to nursing care is to explore the physical, social, environmental, and psychological changes that occur in the older adult and older adults with kidney dysfunction.

C. To provide comprehensive and competent care, the nurse needs to become proficient in blending the multifaceted changes so the older adult can live at an optimal level of health with the most independence that is realistic and possible. This endeavor can and will be a challenge as nurses care for more older adults with the complexities related to AKI and CKD.

References

Adams, M., Holland, L., & Urban, C. (2013). *Pharmacology for nurses: A pathophysiologic approach* (4th ed.). Upper Saddle River, NJ: Prentice Hall.

American Nurses Association (2010). *Scope and standards of gerontological nursing*. Silver Spring, MD: American Nurses Association.

Bowling, C.B., & O'Hare, A.M. (2012). Managing older adults with CKD: Individualized versus disease-based approaches. *American Journal of Kidney Diseases*, 59(2), 293-302.

Brown, E., & Johansson, L. (2010). Broadening options for long-term dialysis in the elderly (BOLDE): Differences in quality of life on peritoneal dialysis compared to hemodialysis for older patients. *Nephrology Dialysis Transplantation*, 25(11), 3755-3763.

Campbell, K.H., Dale, W., Stankus, N., & Sachs, G.A. (2008). Older adults and chronic kidney disease decision-making by primary care physicians: A scholarly review and research agenda. *Journal of General Internal Medicine*, 23(3), 329-336.

Centers for Disease Control and Prevention (CDC). (2010). *Deaths and mortality*. Retrieved from http://www.cdc.gov/nchs/fastats/deaths.htm

Centers for Disease Control and Prevention (CDC). (2011). *Life expectancy*. Retrieved from http://www.cdc.gov/nchs/fastats/life-expectancy.htm

Centers for Disease Control and Prevention (CDC). (2012). *Influenza*. Retrieved from http://www.cdc.gov/flu/about/qa/research.htm

Centers for Medicare and Medicaid Services (CDC). (2014). *Medicare program: General information*. Retrieved from http://www.cms.gov/Medicare/Medicare-General-Information/MedicareGenInfo/index.html

Cheung, C.M., Ponnusamy, A., & Anderton, J.G. (2008). Management of acute renal failure in the elderly patient: A clinician's guide, *Drugs and Aging*, 25(6), 455-476.

Corbin, J. & Strauss, A. (1991). A nursing model for chronic illness management based upon the trajectory framework. *Scholarly Inquiry for Nursing Practice*, 5, 155-174.

Counts, C.S. (Ed.). (2008). *Core curriculum for nephrology nursing*. Pitman, NJ: American Nephrology Nurses' Association.

Curry, R. (2008). Ageism in healthcare: Time for a change. *Aging Well, 1*, 16.

Danaei, G., Rimm, E.B., Oza S., Kulkarni, S.C., Murray, C.J. (2010) *The promise of prevention: The effects of four preventable risk factors on national life expectancy and life expectancy disparities by race and county in the United States.* PLoS Med 7(3), e1000248. doi:10.1371/journal.pmed.1000248

Desai, A.K., Grossbery, G.T., & Chibnall, J.T. (2010). Health brain aging: A road map. *Clinics in Geriatric Medicine, 26*(1), 1-16.

Eliopoulos, C. (2014). *Gerontological nursing* (8th ed.). Philadelphia: Lippincott Williams & Wilkins.

European Dialysis and Transplantation Nurses Association. (2011). *Caring for the elderly renal patient: A guide to clinical practice.* Luzern, Switzerland: EDTNA/ERCA.

Jones, D.S., Podolsky, S.H., & Greene, J.A. (2012). The burden of disease and the changing task of medicine. *New England Journal of Medicine*, 366, 2333-2338. doi:10.1056/NEJMp1113569

Lamping, D.L. (2000). Clinical outcomes, quality of life, and costs in the North Thames Dialysis Study of elderly people on dialysis: A prospective cohort study. *Lancet, 356*, 1543-1550

Lewington, A., & Kanagasundaram, S. (2011). Acute kidney injury. Retrieved from http://www.renal.org/guidelines/modules/acute-kidney-injury#sthash.nxd9dnYv.dpbs

McCance, K. L., Huether, S. E., Brashers, V. L., & Rote, N. S. (2010). *Pathophysiology: The biologic basis for disease in adults and children* (6th ed.). Marilyn Heights, MO: Mosby Elsevier.

Mauk, K.L. (2006). *Gerontological nursing: Competencies for care* (2nd ed.). Burlington, MA: Jones & Bartlett Learning.

National Network for Immunization Information. (2010a). *Influenza.* Retrieved from http://www.immunizationinfo.org/vaccines/influenza#history-of-the-vaccine

National Network for Immunization Information. (2010b). *Pneumococcal.* Retrieved from http://www.immunizationinfo.org/vaccines/pneumococcal-disease

New Jersey Medical School Global Tuberculosis Institute. (2012). *A history of tuberculosis treatment.* Retrieved from http://www.umdnj.edu/ntbcweb/tbhistory.htm

Planton, J. & Edluna, B.J. (2010). Strategies for reducing poly-pharmacy in older adults. *Journal of Gerontologic Nursing, 36*, 8.

Samiy, A.H. (1983). Renal disease in the elderly: Treatment options. *Medical Clinics of North America, 67*(2), 463-480.

Tablowski, P. A. (2014). *Gerontological nursing* (3rd ed.) Upper Saddle River, NJ: Pearson Education, Inc.

Touhy, T.A., & Jett, K. (2012). *Ebersole & Hess' toward healthy aging: Human needs nursing response* (8th ed.). St. Louis: Mosby Elsevier.

United States Census Bureau. (2010). *The 2010 statistical abstract.* Retrieved from http://www.census.gov/compendia/statab/

United States Census Bureau. (2011). *The older population: 2010.* Retrieved from http://www.census.gov/prod/cen2010/briefs/c2010br-09.pdf

United States Department of Health and Human Services Administration on Aging. (2010). *Projected future growth of the older population.* Retrieved from http://www.aoa.gov/Aging_Statistics/future_growth/future_growth.aspx#age

United States Department of Health and Human Services. (2011). *Health, United States, 2011.* Retrieved from http://www.cdc.gov/nchs/data/hus/hus11.pdf#022

United States Renal Data System. (2012). 2012 *Annual data report: Atlas of chronic kidney disease and end-stage renal disease in the United States.* Retrieved from http://www.usrds.org/adr.aspx

United States Renal Data System. (2014). *CKD in the general population.* Retrieved from http://www.usrds.org/2014/view/v1_01.aspx

Weiss, J. W., Petrik, A. F., & Thorp, M. L. (2011). Identification and management of chronic kidney disease in older adults. *Clinical Geriatrics, 19*(2), 33-37.

Woog, P. (Ed.). (1992). The chronic illness trajectory: *The Corbin and Strauss nursing model.* New York: Springer.

Appendix 2.1. Systemic Age-Related Changes and Implications

System	Age-Related Changes and Implications
Integument	Decrease in eccrine, apocrine, and sebaceous glands leading to skin dryness.
	Decrease in number of melanocytes leading to decreased photoprotection.
	Adipose tissue redistributes and leads to increased adipose tissue in waistline and hips.
	Decreased touch receptors; slowing of reflexes and pain sensation.
	Increased probability of pressure ulcers due to decreased blood flow and thinner .
	Decreased elasticity with decreased tensile strength.
	Hair thins and turns gray.
	Decreased elastin and development of wrinkles.
	Loss of eyelid elasticity.
Respiratory	Atrophy of the muscles of respiration and structural changes of the rib cage inhibit movement and lung inflation, resulting in decreased vital capacity, increased residual capacity, and increased dead space. This results in diminished lung sounds, especially at the base.
	Reductions in lung volume and capacity cause the older adult to use more physical energy to breathe.
	Decreased cilia and cough result in decreased mucous and airway clearance, causing the elderly to be at increased risk for infection.
	Decreased numbers of alveoli.
	Decreased response to hypercapnia. Arterial hypoxemia with reduced PO_2 levels.
	Calcification of costal makes the trachea and rib cage more rigid.
	The anterior-posterior diameter increases, often demonstrated by kyphosis.
	Thoracic inspiratory and expiratory muscles are weaker.
	Alveoli become flatter and shallower and there is a decrease in the amount of tissue dividing individual alveoli. There is a decrease in surface area (decreased gas exchange).
	The lungs become smaller and more rigid and have less recoil.
	The lungs exhale less effectively.
	If respiratory activity is reduced under normal circumstances, one can imagine the profound effects of immobility on the respiratory system.
	The diaphragm may weaken up to 25%, limiting respirations.

Continues on next page

System	Age-Related Changes and Implications
Musculoskeletal	Loss of lean body mass (sarcopenia) causes a decrease in muscle strength.
	Decreased testosterone can lead to an increase in bone loss and declining muscle mass and strength.
	Decreased estrogen in women leads to increased bone loss and development of osteoporosis.
	Loss of bone structure and density and deterioration of cartilage in joints result in increased risk of fractures and limitation of range of motion.
	Increased porosity of the bone reduces the strength of the bone.
	Decreased osteoblastic activity increases the risk for fractures and prolongs the time for bone healing.
	Thinning of intervertebral disks and compression of vertebral bodies lead to a loss of stature.
	Decreased elasticity of tendons and ligaments leads to altered gait, impaired mobility, and increased risk for falls.
	The joint capsule and ligaments become shorter, stiffer, and less able to stretch.
	Cartilage lining the bones becomes calcified, thinner, and less resilient. As a result, it becomes more difficult to move, and range of motion is reduced.
	Initiation and speed of movement begins to slow with age. Slower reaction time.
Nervous	Decreased number of neurons with accumulation of senile plaques and neurofibrillary tangles.
	Decrease in brain size and weight.
	Decreased blood flow to the brain.
	Decrease in short-term memory.
	Increased incidence of benign senescence.
	Increase reaction time and slowed responses.
	Increased pain threshold.
	Insomnia and other sleep disturbances increase, including loss of REM sleep that may result in daytime fatigue and instability.
	Deep tendon reflexes may be absent in some older adults.
	Depression and mood disorders become more common.
	Decreased sensation to light touch, pain, and joint position.
Immune	Decreased antibody production; increased risk for infection, delayed healing, and slowing recovery from illness.
	Reduced antibody production with increased risk for developing an infection or disease reactivation.
	Atrophy of the thymus gland leads to lack of T-cell differentiation, causing the body to attack itself.
	Decreased fever response.
	Delayed or decreased hypersensitivity response as evidenced by milder reactions to TB testing.
	Decreased ability to exhibit an inflammatory response.
	Reduced antigen response.
	Increased autoantibody production – increased risk for autoimmune disease such as rheumatoid

Continues on next page

System	Age-Related Changes and Implications
Gastrointestinal	Loss of periostal and periodontal bone and gingival retraction cause tooth loss and reduced ability to masticate.
	Production of saliva decreases (dry mouth), and reduced muscles for mastication cause dry mouth and difficulty swallowing.
	Decreased number of taste buds decrease accurate receptors for salt and sweet (hypoguesia).
	Gag reflex is decreased and older adult is at risk for aspiration.
	Cardiac sphincter loses integrity and may cause indigestion, reflux, and hiatal hernia.
	Stomach motility and emptying are reduced (feelings of fullness, heartburn, and indigestion).
	Decreased gastric secretions result in diminished absorption of calcium, Vitamin B12, and folic acid.
	Both large and small intestines have some atrophy; with decreased peristalsis, constipation and abdominal discomfort.
	Weakened intestinal walls can lead to diverticular disease.
	Decline in bile acid synthesis can result in gallstones.
	The liver decreases in weight and storage capacity. There is also a decrease in pancreatic enzymes. All of these factors can result in decreased drug metabolism and an increased risk for drug toxicity.
Sensory	Conduction disturbances, sensory and neural deteriorations, changes in thickness of tympanic membrane, and hair cell loss lead to loss of hearing high-frequency tones (presbycusis) and cause difficulty understanding speech or filtering out background noise.
	Increased production and accumulation of dry cerumen cause decreased hearing abilities.
	Declines in vestibular function in the inner ear can cause alterations in equilibrium and balance.
	Decreased number of olfactory neurons can lead to diminished ability to sense odors.
	Rigidity of the eye lens and decreased accommodation cause difficulty focusing on near objects (presbyopia) and impair reading abilities.
	Diminished lacrimation leads to "dry eyes."
	Decreased pupil size alters the amount of light to the retina and causes a reduced field of vision. Night vision is reduced.
	Increased particles in the vitreous humor cause "floaters" in the visual field.
	Increased intraocular pressure results in glaucoma.
	Decreased ability to adjust to changes in light intensity.
	Age-Related Eye Diseases
	Cataracts A decrease in the transparency of the lens of the eye. Lens become cloudy and vision is blurred.
	Glaucoma Increased intraocular pressure secondary to an abnormal buildup of aqueous humor in the eye. Causes loss of peripheral vision. Diminished vision in dim light.
	Macular degeneration Gradual loss of central vision. Distorted straight lines. Blurred vision.

Continues on next page

System	Age-Related Changes and Implications
Endocrine	Decreased secretion of insulin increasing risk for developing diabetes mellitus Type II.
	Decreased sensitivity to insulin resulting in a variation of blood glucose levels.
	Peripheral tissues may become insulin resistant, especially in the presence of obesity.
	Loss of circadian rhythm of antidiuretic hormone secretion leading to increased nocturnal urine production.
	Reduced secretion of aldosterone.
	Reduced secretion of renin.
	Reduced secretion of angiotensin.
	Increased atrial natriuretic peptide levels.
Cardiovascular	Heart size does not change significantly with age. Enlarged hearts are associated with cardiac disease.
	Arterial stiffening contributes to decline in peripheral and vital organ perfusion. Some peripheral pulses may not be palpable.
	Veins thicken and valvular reflux (secondary to valve incompetence) contributes to varicosities. Dependent edema can occur with long periods of sitting without elevating feet.
	AV valves become thick and rigid, a result of sclerosis and fibrosis.
	The heart muscle loses its efficiency and contractile strength, resulting in reduction in cardiac output under conditions of physiologic stress.
	There is increased electrical irregularity secondary to a decrease in the number of pacemaker cells and a thickening of the shell surrounding the sinus node (increased risk for atrial fibrillation and other dysrthymias).
	Decreased elasticity of the arteries is responsible for vascular changes in heart and kidney.
	Decrease in sensitivity of baroreceptors can result in postural hypotension.
	Older adults gradually notice changes in the cardiovascular system. These age-related changes are most apparent when unusual demands are placed on the heart (e.g., shoveling snow).
	Mental status changes, agitation, and falls may be the first signs of cardiac problems in the older person.
Hematologic	Decline in active bone marrow with reduced ability to accelerate RBC production.
	Neutrophil and monocyte activity decreases but WBC remains relatively stable.
	Platelet adhesion may increase with corresponding increases in fibrinogen and clotting factors.
	Total serum iron, iron binding capacity, and intestinal iron absorption are decreased with potential for iron deficiency anemia.

Continues on next page

System	Age-Related Changes and Implications
Urinary	Decreased estrogen and pelvic relaxation can cause stress incontinence and an overactive bladder.
	Bladder capacity decreases, and the micturition reflex is delayed.
	Hyperplasia and hypertrophy of the prostate in men can result in difficulty urinating and urge incontinence.
	Increase in nocturia or increase in number of fluid voids at night leading to sleep disturbance.
	Decreased bladder contractility secondary to weakening and thinning of the detrusor smooth muscle.
	Detrusor instability leading to incontinence.
	Decreased bladder capacity by about 50%.
	Inability to concentrate urine with increased risk for dehydration.
	Decreased sensation of bladder fullness resulting in less frequent voiding.
	Potential for overflow incontinence and urinary retention in men.
Renal	Decreased blood flow to kidneys secondary to atrophy of the supply blood vessels.
	Decline in kidney function including filtration rate and prolonged half-life of drugs.
	Increased kidney threshold for glucose.
	Decline in kidney mass, primarily from the cortex.
	Focal glomerulosclerosis predisposing to loss of nephrons.
Reproductive	**Males**
	Testosterone decreases leading to erectile dysfunction.
	Sperm count decreases but production never ceases.
	Testes decrease in size and weight.
	Length of time to achieve an erection increases (fibrosis in erectile tissue) ; erection becomes less full.
	Require more stimulation in order to maintain the erection.
	Usually experience less intense orgasms, and ejaculation decreases in ejaculatory volume.
	Prostatic enlargement.
	Females
	Elasticity of pelvic area decreased; increased risk for uterine/vaginal prolapsed.
	Ovaries atrophy and number of ovarian follicles decrease with age. By age 50–65, there are no remaining viable follicles.
	Estrogen and progesterone levels decrease leading to menopause.
	Breast tissue decreases.
	Uterus atrophies and size decreases about 50%.
	Vagina becomes shorter and narrower.
	Vaginal walls become thinner with less elasticity.
	Vaginal lubrication decreases leading to painful intercourse.
	Vaginal secretions become alkaline- increased risk for vaginal infections.
	Labia majora shrinks and becomes separated. May increase risk for infections (greater surface area exposed).
	Decreased estrogen can cause vaginal dryness, vaginal atrophy, and decreased size of the ovaries and uterus.

Adapted from K. L. Mauk (2006). *Gerontological nursing: Competencies for care*. Copyright 2006 by Jones and Bartlett.

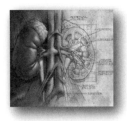

SELF-ASSESSMENT QUESTIONS FOR MODULE 5

These questions apply to all chapters in Module 5 and can be used for self-testing. They are not considered part of the official CNE process.

Chapter 1

1. Symptoms that would be expected in a child with cystinosis would be which of the following?
   a. Oliguria.
   b. Anorexia.
   c. Lack of growth.
   d. Splenomegaly.

2. Psychosocial impacts on parents of children diagnosed with CKD include which of the following (select all that apply)?
   a. Depression as there is no cure.
   b. Fear of treatment modalities.
   c. Energy spent on working to afford the bills.
   d. Plans for children's future changing.

3. Common causes of acute kidney failure include all the following except
   a. liver failure.
   b. NSAIDs.
   c. urethral obstruction.
   d. hypervolemia.

4. The **two** specific needs of pediatric patients using hemodialysis as a treatment modality are (choose two)
   a. fluid removal to prevent long-term complications.
   b. developmental and socialization efforts.
   c. the length of time required to spend in the center.
   d. emotional response to the cause of the kidney failure.

5. Challenges to caring for pediatric individuals receiving CRRT are (choose all that apply)
   a. nutrition.
   b. growth.
   c. hormonal impacts.
   d. body image issues.

6. Methods of providing supplemental nutrition to children with CKD would include
   a. jejunal or duodenal tube feedings.
   b. increased protein in milk shake form.
   c. encouraging the child to eat whatever they want.
   d. providing vegetables in pureed form.

Chapter 2

7. In 1900, the primary causes of death were related to _____; however, in 2010, the primary causes of death were directly related to _____
   a. infectious diseases, lifestyle choices.
   b. lifestyle choices, infectious disease.

8. Which of the following occurs because of a normal physiologic change in the immune system of an older adult?
   a. Increased antibody production.
   b. Increased risk for development of infections.
   c. Increased ability to exhibit an inflammatory response.
   d. Increased antigen response.

9. On average, how many different medications will the non-institutionalized older adult take routinely?
   a. 1–4.
   b. 5–7.
   c. 8–13.
   d. 14–17.

10. With an increase in the older adult population and the simultaneous increase in the number of older adults diagnosed with CKD, Medicare expenditures will also increase. According to the USRDS (2012), Medicare expenditures for older adults with CKD comprised _____ of the total Medicare funds.
    a. 10%.
    b. 17%.
    c. 25%.
    d. 33%.

11. Which of the following complexities of providing care to the older adult with CKD can have a direct effect on developing the treatment regimen?
    a. Functional loss.
    b. Cognitive impairment.
    c. Comorbidities.
    d. All of the above.

12. What is the advantage of an older adult choosing peritoneal dialysis as a treatment modality vs. hemodialysis?
    a. Fluids are removed faster with peritoneal dialysis.
    b. Solutes are removed faster with peritoneal dialysis.
    c. Risk of transmission of viral diseases is reduced.
    d. Risk of transmission of bacterial infections is reduced.

Answer Key

Chapter 1		Chapter 2	
1.	c	7.	a
2.	a, b, c	8.	b
3.	d	9.	c
4.	a and b	10.	b
5.	a, b, c, d	11.	d
6.	a	12.	c

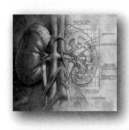

INDEX FOR MODULE 5

Page numbers followed by **f** indicate figures.
Page numbers followed by **t** indicate tables

Core Curriculum for Nephrology Nursing, Sixth Edition © 2015 American Nephrology Nurses' Association